INTUITIVE EATING

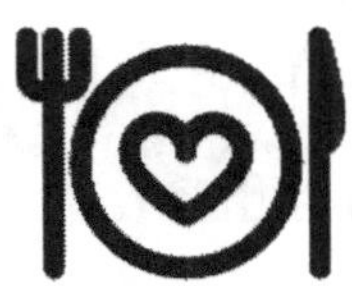

AN EFFECTIVE ANTI-DIET GUIDE TO
RESTORING A HAPPY RELATIONSHIP WITH
FOOD, FREE YOURSELF FROM DIETING,
REACH FOREVER YOUR HEALTHY WEIGHT,
SLOW DOWN YOUR AGING PROCESS

Evelyn Dooner

This book shows a simple secret to lose weight by eating your preferred food.

It's far from the numerous diets all over the world

"Eating is necessity, healthy eating is an art"

François de la Rochefoucauld

TABLE OF CONTENTS

INTRODUCTION 9

   L.W.B.E 9

   AN INCREDIBLE STORY 13

   THE SOCIAL IMPACT OF FOOD COMPANIES 17

Chapter 1

THE FIRST STEPS TO DISCOVER THIS EXCLUSIVE FOOD EDUCATION 21

Chapter 2

HOW TO SLOW DOWN THE PACE OF YOUR LIFE AND PREPARE YOURSELF TO CHANGE MINDSET AND EATING HABITS 26

   " A Healthy Mind In A Healthy Body " 29

Chapter 3

THE SECRET TO NEVER BEING ON A DIET AGAIN AND REACHING YOUR HEALTHY WEIGHT WITHOUT SUFFERING 34

Chapter 4

LEARN QUICKLY AND EASILY HOW TO PRACTICE THE SECRET 39

Chapter 5

HOW TO TREAT YOUR MEALTIME 47

Chapter 6

THE FOUR ESSENTIAL NUTRITIONAL SUPPLEMENTS
FOR GUARANTEED RESULTS 52

Chapter 7

HOW TO OVERCOME HUNGER WITHOUT COMMITMENT
AND SUFFERING 59

Chapter 8

YOUR GREATEST ALLY AND HOW TO TAKE ADVANTAGE
OF IT DURING THE FIRST MONTH.............. 64

THE ACTIONS TO MAKE THIS FIRST MONTH 73

Chapter 9

ONE OF THE MOST IMPORTANT ESSENTIAL FOODS......75

Chapter 10

HOW TO TAKE BACK CONTROL OF YOUR BODY 85

Chapter 11

YOUR EASY 10-WEEK WORK PLAN.................................... 99

Chapter 12

YOUR BEST FOOD COMBINATIONS..................................103

Chapter 13

WHAT YOU SHOULD AVOID LIKE THE PLAGUE.... 114

Chapter 14

DON'T EAT LESS, EAT CONSCIOUSLY! ... AND HOW TO
DO IT 128

EAT RIGHT FOR YOUR BLOOD TYPE........................... 130

Group A Type 131
Group B Type 131
Group AB Type 131
Group O Type 135

Chapter 15

ADVICE TO CHANGE YOUR ERRONEOUS HABITS.........147

Chapter 16

SILENCE IS GOLD ! 152

CONCLUSION..157

Thank You For Reading My Book! 161

"I have a very simple taste,
I'm always satisfied with the best"

Oscar Wilde

INTRODUCTION

L.W.B.E

With this book I will teach you an alimentary system based on simple studies that I started more than 30 years ago. I deal with the topic in a clear, simple, and direct way by using often only subject-verb and object complement. The reader can understand and remember the most important points to learn and practice easily. There are few scientific quotes, recipes, chemical, and organic explanations, but there are only simple suggestions to live and make them personal.

The topics covered in this book can be found in books, in paper articles, and on the internet widely documented.

Meanwhile, this book explains practical and precise strategies to learn to lose weight by eating. The goal of these strategies is to lose weight by eating without restrictions.

We' ll talk mainly about the creation of a diet, a new way to eat that will allow our body to be fed in the best way possible, to lose adipose tissues, and reach the right weight form. To find out this data is enough to do a simple mathematics calculation: You must deduct the first number to body height, in meters (or ft). For example:

a man 1.75 m tall (5.74 ft): if you remove the first number, his optimum weight will be around 75 kg (165.35 lb)... women have lower body mass, so you have to consider that to deduct another 5 /10 kilos (11/22 lb) according to their tiny or junoesque body.

This is a simple calculation to perform to get a long term goal; then, we need to create a track that will bring us to the optimum weight step by step. It will be useless to have time goals that will create performance anxiety removing unnecessary inner peace. This is not very constructive.

This book will stimulate your intellect to get the method and put it into practice. In the next pages, we'll call this system with **LWBE** initials (Lose Weight by Eating).

The secret is in the heart of the book; it will bring you to the right weight and will make you very happy. By engaging oneself, this method is reliable and foolproof. You'll find some rules and suggestions that will help you to practice the LWBE, to allow it to express its potential at its best.

Which is the hard and ruthless truth? Why do you want to change?

Because we are fat, out of shape.

Because we are unhappy inside.

Because for many years, we made wrong choices, years of stress, overwork ourselves, forced inactive, and so on. These reflections don't mean negativity. They represent our reality:

the pure truth. Our society is quietly dangerous and subjects us to conditions and potentially serious poisons. That can undermine our health, and they let us loose our figure easily.

Listen carefully to these words: our society is responsible for our modern world, which is created by companies based only on mere profit at our expense.

The fault is in the message they try to instill in us each day, it's based on - Buy, use and throw it as quickly as possible -, and start over again. This "diktat" influences the alimentary market very much because it concerns a primary need. Buy, use, and throw.

Companies and multinational decentralize millions of dollars for social studies and marketing strategies, to force us to eat their jungle food. Finally, we are easy prey. Sixty years ago, everything was easier and human; life was less dangerous. We ate to live, we were thanking God for all he provides us, there were few fat people. The population was protected from cholesterol, diabetes, heart diseases, and those related to obesity. Hunger belonged only to a few poor families; providence gave healthy food in the right quantities to all the others. Food often was grown or grows naturally.

You must think that the poor diet of the family of that time overlaps perfectly to the alimentary pyramid well known as the perfect way of eating.

Our best nutritionists spent millions of dollars for researches and 30 years to create it; a phone call to their grandparents and taking some notes would have been enough. Diet is based on many seasonal vegetables and fruits, following the level of the pyramid, we find whole cereals and oil, pulses, dried fruit, poultry, eggs and cheese, meta and complex cereals, such as flour and rice. Last rule: daily physical activity and right intake of water.

It seems incredible: This is the picture of our society until the 70s. In very little time, we reached an unrecognizable world from all points of view, strange confused overwhelming and swiftly, where there is too much of everything. Once there was bread, now, if you get into a supermarket there are twenty different kinds of bread. You find dozen and dozen of water bottles that come from the most unimaginable places. Sparkling natural water and even "foreign" water; if we talk about wines, fries, candies, or biscuits, we reach the ridge of the ridge in quantity. Let's think about the many useless sold beverages. In US supermarkets there are 30 meters (98 ft) of lanes and five shelves with different kinds of corn flakes or orange drinks. some American malls are so huge that they put electric cars to their clients to let them move around. The word that rules the world is: too much. We take away to the third world too much, Too much is what makes us vulnerable both from psychological and physical aspects.

Let's stop for a second and look around.

How many useless sophisticated and less human things are around us. They deprive us of social relationships and love that is what we need.

We fill up this lack of love, by focusing our attention on all our basic needs, such as eating. Media draws our attention constantly on useless and unhealthy products. The majority of food that reaches our tables is treated with preservatives, sweeteners, dyestuffs, and natural flavors. The most interesting example is fast food.

We are the subject of sleek scientific and marketing studies. They convince us to buy products made to create addiction; all this produces billions of dollars turnover with serious consequences. All over the world. In consumerism, what scandalizes mostly is waste. Mother Theresa of Calcutta said: One-third of produced food goes into the garbage. Imagine how much food was produced today, one part of three ends up in the trash. We'll talk again about it further.

AN INCREDIBLE STORY

I would like to tell you Morgan Spurlok's story, a hero of our times.

In the Year 2004 he wanted to prove the danger of sophisticated food made specifically for consumers, to make them dependent on this alimentary brand.

Spurlok's dramatic documentary gives us a perfect idea of how they want to manipulate our conscience.

I would like to underline a very important thing: the experiment concerns fast food, but it could have the same result with different categories of food. Everything started in a new report in the year 2002. A couple of American girls sued a popular fast-food chain; it was the guilt of their obesity. The company's legal office bet on the fact that there were no proofs and that feeding principally based on their products was healthy. They won the lawsuit!

Spurlok was a writer and a well-known TV producer. He wanted to prove precisely the contrary to what was stated by the law sentence. He decided to eat only food in that chain for one month. He documented this experience by 24 hours camera. In the beginning, Morgan did a check-up with three doctors: a generic doctor, a cardiologist, and a gastroenterologist. They monitored him during this time. They declared he was perfectly healthy on average, he was a sportsman, 1.84 tall (6 ft) and his weight was 84 kilos (185 lb). They expressed him would have had bad effects on his body for sure: they expected a moderate weight gain and an increase of cholesterol rate, but none of then expected such a drastic result. One of the doctors claimed the human body is suitable for all kinds of food.

Spurlok started with breakfast in a fast food joint in Manhattan, his town of birth. You can find a fast food joint every 0.7 km (0.43 mi) there. He moved only by taxi, reducing daily walk steps to about 2500 steps, the average of an American man. There were precise, common, and strict rules to follow during the experiment, as far as the dietary attitude concerns.

He must have 3 meals a day in that fast food.

He must eat every menu option each time

He must order only meals that are on the menu

He must accept to take the supersize menu if proposed from waiters.

The second day Morgan ate the super menu, and he had his first stomach ache as well as nausea. 5 days later, he gained 5 kilos (11 lb). After a couple of days, he was depressed, his depression and headache subsided only by eating another meal in that fast food.

One of the three doctors that took care of him thought he became dependent. He lost 500 grams (1.10 lb) at a certain point, but after a while, he gained 5 kilos (11 lb) reaching 92 kilos (202.83 lb) of weight. He later gained 11 kilos (24.25 lb). Spurlok put on weight almost half a kilo (1.10 lb) each day.

Once the experiment ended, he took 6 months to come back to his initial weight. His wife Alexandra Jamieson, a popular vegetarian chef, helped him to detoxify with an appropriate strict diet. She confirmed that he lost a lot of his energy and libido during this experiment.

After 20 days he had a tachycardia episode. Doctor Daryl Isaac, one of his 3 doctors, declared these textual words: his liver is becoming a melted paste. He asked him to stop the experiment to avoid serious heart problems. He was compared to the leading actor of "**Leaving Las Vegas**": He drinks advisedly for a similar period until he died.

Morgan changed some of the diets, and he continued to follow the imposed rules.

He ate more salad but in fast food, it has a great quantity of sugar. He reached his goal: and was obese on the 30th day.

All three doctors were surprised by his health deterioration. Beside personal troubles, different factors that let the USA have the highest rate of obesity were investigated in the documentary:

The lack of healthy food in many American schools and the negative power of advertisements on young people were investigated.

THE SOCIAL IMPACT OF FOOD COMPANIES

There are many examples of this kind of concern towards human beings from food companies. The majority of them are not known and hidden, unfortunately, they often affect young people.

The good is that with the LWBE system we will handle all this food and we'll win.

The secret works so well that you can eat mildly, also in fast-food chains without any problems.

Our usual way of eating, that I define real food consumerism, creates real paradoxes. Food that is produced a few kilometers from us and you can buy from your house, are often refused in favor of products produced very far, they cost more, and their quality is not certain.

Food cultivated and produced near us is called "zero kilometers". This means it's controlled, it's very fresh and cheaper because it has a short distance to reach us. Many times we eat tomatoes that taste of water while the zero kilometer counterparts are juicy and very good. They are tomatoes that taste of tomatoes.

Here's an example:

Companies that handle water made massive TV advertisements. They invent all that is possible. Their sources are in different locations. Now, this is a very simple question: If I should import water from several hundred miles, who is going to pay the fuel for the trucks? How much pollution is created from transportation? How much money will it cost to transport these bottles for such a long trip?

How many millions are spent on advertisements that will affect the price of each bottle?

Recall we used to drink water from taps. Nowadays, due to strict laws about the potability of flowing water, in many cases, I'm sure that the water which flows from taps is better than many advertised water brands, at most it's enough to add some baking soda, if the flavor is not good to your taste, you can use the filter pitchers that you find on the market. Furthermore, all this exaggerated variety of products found in supermarkets have an expiring date, food is thrown in the garbage, and its cost is amortized in sales.

This is a double abuse. We buy a box paying all possible and imaginable costs, from poisoning fertilizer to the well-calculated final percentage of packs that will be sent to waste because they'll expire before they are consumed. As we said before 1/3 of the food we produce each day goes in the garbage. 1/3 of food in our evolved world is very much, very very much! One bread piece out of 3 goes to garbage. It will be enough to feed most poor countries in the third world each year.

Though we can escape from this vicious, dramatic, and terrible circle.

This little examples should make you understand that we are led from consumerism and are so suited to that to think that it's our real life.

LWBE can help you to escape from this slavery and return to wellness and ideal weight.

The title of this book is: "Intuitive Eating" because it allows you to eat what you want, and it will lead you to choose the right food, and you will see that you'll always choose the best ones!

"The most charming show on the earth is a beautiful woman cooking for the one she loves."

Tom Wolf

Chapter 1

THE FIRST STEPS TO DISCOVER THIS EXCLUSIVE FOOD EDUCATION

The first essential duty is to go to the doctor and ask for a complete check-up. This will allow you to know your health state, and to start in the best way possible.

It might be that, there are values out of the normal to be rebalanced. To have wrong data, could compromise the formation of the new diet and its use during the time.

You should do:

-Blood and thyroid test

-To control if you're affected by celiac disease

-Find out your blood group

-Find out if there are some intolerances and allergies

Furthermore, control your fat mass, height, and weight so that you will have basic data to measure your progress. You should avoid everything that can compromise the LWBE in the body, without your knowledge. You should ensure that a full check-up is done at least once a year or a maximum of two years. Prevention is better than to treat. It will be the best money spent in your life. Then you should choose a day and start!

Planning will prepare you psychologically to start a change, to start afresh.

If I should suggest a period to prepare, I'll say one month at least. During this time, you can concentrate and start to study how to personalize the rules of LWBE; you can solve a physical and operational problem, for example, to conform yourself to deducted restrictions from medical exams. On the other hand, you will have time to discover quality foods. In thirty days, you'll have enough time to organize yourself to do some researches and to proof and practice the different rules that you will learn.

This work will be handy for the future. Take your time to start by avoiding phase or physical goals.

Now it's time to go slowly to adjust. It's time to start to love your body and your soul; you need time to rediscover yourself. It's very important to understand that you are building a diet, and this is very far from a slimming diet. This is not your typical nightmare that lasts one, two, three; six months, and then you will end up worse than before. The classic life of a diet ". It's called "yo-yo life" (from the game) because you gain weight and you lose it, to gain it one more time. This is terrible.

Soul-destroying!

How many diets have you tried?

How much did you suffer?

How much money did you spend?

What were your results?

Alimentary diet is fulfilling and lasts a lifetime; its goal is to change our relationship with food and create new attitudes to feel good and eat right. This means to allow our body to come back to ideal weight without food deprivations, but it acts only on the way we eat. We learned many negative habits and now we eat unhealthily. Results are that we easily gain weight without knowing how it happened. We feel depressed, and we do not know how to solve this problem. We say that we should start a diet but then we postponed it or are not able even to start. Sometimes, the required sacrifices compared to obtained results discourage us, so we lose our self-confidence, and quit.

The main cause of that is our society with its strong and conflicting messages. Milliard dollars are spent on marketing and ads informing us that for one to be slim you must buy certain products but then, you must go to the gym and to the doctor to lose weight. On the other hand, millions are spent to convince you to eat junk food and to become a slave of it happily.

Let's try to explain to a poor African child: we eat too much, so, we need a place to run, we lift weight to loose what is too much for the body. Others eat so much that they visit a doctor who tells them what to do to lose weight. But only a few can do it, others stay fat. imagine telling a poor child: "you there, little child, what are you doing?" I'm hungry.

It's dramatic that we have such a huge difference between us and the third world. The leader of nations could solve the problem of hunger in the world very easily. Unfortunately, the consciences of the big ones think to themselves by neglecting the poor. Do you know what is worse? These strategies are used in all modern consumerism fields.

Let's go back to our alimentary program. We're creating a diet: so do not hurry. To change an attitude you need at least a month, if you try to shorten this period, you will work in wrongly and hastily; if you are superficial to respect the classic thirty-day rule, you'll develop a fragile LWBE plan, full of gaps in the long run. You should take time for each step, allow it to become a habit; then, it will happen automatically without even realizing it. The joy that LWBE will give you will help to apply yourself daily, with always more love towards you. The results will come early very early. They'll be tangible from the first weeks.

Chapter 2

HOW TO SLOW DOWN THE PACE OF YOUR LIFE AND PREPARE YOURSELF TO CHANGE MINDSET AND EATING HABITS

Now, while you're practicing the change of your wrong attitudes that are rooted in your life for many years, you should move with kindness and patience; it will be enough to follow the secrets and rules, and your body will automatically acquire them.

For example, the first day you start to drink the famous two liters of water, recommended by doctors to have perfect body hydration and excellent fitness, within a week, **the body will drown in water.** It will be too much for your body, and it will refuse it. If you start by increasing by say half a glass daily, after twenty days, you will achieve that goal. Resign yourself, two liters per day. It's impossible to even for who invented it. One and half-liter are enough, you will get more quantity with food and other sources. Remember to be rational and gentle with yourself.

The LWBE has its fundamental sentence:

*" **With Kindness You Get Everything** "*

This is an essential alimentary diet that tries to make our lives better in all aspects.

To do this, you should consider yourself as a 5-year-old child that must learn slowly, without pressures, avoiding competitions and goals.

Be kind and positive to yourself, it's all you have. It's the very beginning so you can have some satisfaction too. If you feel like eating a piece of chocolate, eat it. Let it melt in your mouth. To overstress with privations could be worse.

If you abandon chocolate suddenly, it means that each time you see it, you'll bite your lips, and you become nervous which will be worse than abstinence. You will be anxious and you will desire it much more. On the other hand, allow yourself some pleasures. Sure it will be exaggerated to eat a whole piece, but it's only a piece of chocolate, and it's allowed in LWBE. If you eat in the right way, you can eat chocolate all your life, together with other culinary delights.

I eat half a piece each day, and I'm in perfect ideal weight: I'm greedy and happy. The body and mind need gratifications in all fields of life, above all, in daily nutrition. Unfortunately, there were nutritional changes these last decades, that increase the number of food products, but the quality has reduced and consequently the satisfaction they give. As I already said about fast food: flavors are very good, but it's only chemistry and junk food. The mind is practically forced to eat junk food that the body will refuse. To practice LWBE is a gradual process; the body will start to talk to you kindly. It did before, but we were focused on eating junk foods and never listened to the signs. The body and mind will get better slowly with our alimentary diet. We will feel happier, stronger, and full of energy, it will get easier as you go on. You'll get back happiness, and it will grow more and more.

Remember what they say:

" *A Healthy Mind In A Healthy Body* "

translated in latin, the language of the ancient Romans:

" *Mens Sana In Corpore Sano* "

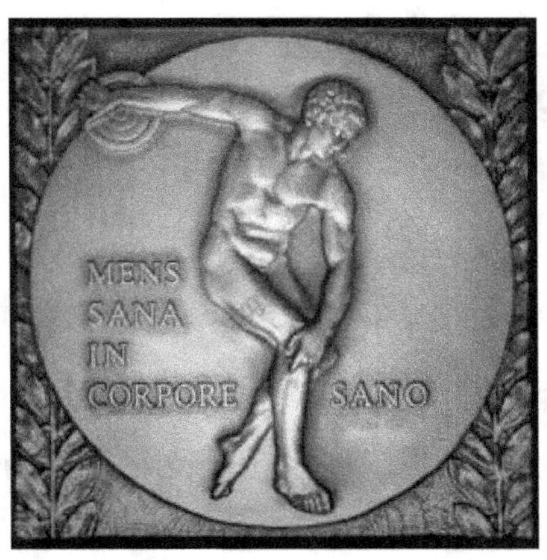

This is another very important factor: <u>the quality of rest</u>.

Intellect and thoughtfulness should work together here. It is essential to sleep in the best way is possible by adopting all the strategies on how to sleep properly. You should give importance to the sleep-waking cycle, as much as drinking water or breathing properly. Sleeping well is very important. Sleeping could be interrupted only if we make love, otherwise engage yourself to have excellent sleep quality. One hundred years ago, there were candles. At sunset people use to gather together around a fireplace, people relaxed and then slept. In the morning, some cocks woke us up, and the day has begun. The brain is at 100%, energy at its maximum. Nowadays? Let's see how we live the night or rest today. The quality is bad under all points of view. Each night we go to bed at different times.

Often, we end the day in front of a computer or "great" television. Watch our life with the last huge fashion of the moment. Chat, artificial lights confuse our rest- wake rhythm. It's wrong to demonize all these achievements of humanity. Though we must handle them with intellect, consciously, without being slaves to them. I would like to talk to you about a particular discovery I made some years back. Everyone knows Ibiza, the famous happy isle of Bale in south Spain. Vacation times are peculiar here. Tourists normally go out of the house at midnight, they have dinner, they go to a disco to spend some time enjoying with others. As usual, nights pass happily until the first lights of the day. At that time all discos shut off and tourists reach a disco that opens at 7:30. 7:30, the Disco stuff has just got up, and it is fresh and lucid in mind, such as a bank employee or a barman of a cafe along the seaside. Then tourists sleep some hours and wake up around 1 pm. They have breakfast, and they go down the shore until 6 pm. They take a shower, and they go to bed again. They wake up at midnight to have dinner, and they go to the disco only coming back to bad at 9 -10 in the morning. Crazy! Thank god they go on vacation once in a year! The most ridiculous thing is that: my husband and I used to go to the beach around 9; we were awake and full of energy.

We went back at 1 pm to eat, and then we take a nap in the afternoon. We go back to the beach at 4.pm. Then we have appetizer and dinner; after dinner, a short walk, and we sleep from exhaustion, we went to bed maximum at midnight. Practically, we were awake when everybody was asleep, and we saw a few people around. We lived in Ibiza (a Spanish island) for 15 days as a quiet isle of palms lost in the "Pacific Ocean." This is only a paradoxical example, but it makes you think very much about how this trend affects the quality of sleep. If it's ten in the night and you are sleepy, go to bed. This is a sane attitude that will help your life because it is positive. Your life will change completely, if you lay down in your soft and cozy bed, at certain times, early in the night. This will help you to get the best from LWBE. Socrates said that after sunset it's better to make only friendly and soft speeches because the brain will continue to work, with complicated and philosophical arguments, also during the night; you will wake up more tired than before. We have books, computers, and televisions. They are useful and positive instruments but let's pay attention, we have to control them based on our necessity.

To make a summary of this chapter: You must love yourself. Face the changes with kindness and pay attention to your rest.

This first month must learn to do our activities with more kindness, love, and passion and to organize oneself to go to bed before 11 pm each day.

"I have no doubt there is a more shocking surprise in the world than the first time you taste an ice cream".

Heywood Campbell Broun

Chapter 3

THE SECRET TO NEVER BEING ON A DIET AGAIN AND REACHING YOUR HEALTHY WEIGHT WITHOUT SUFFERING

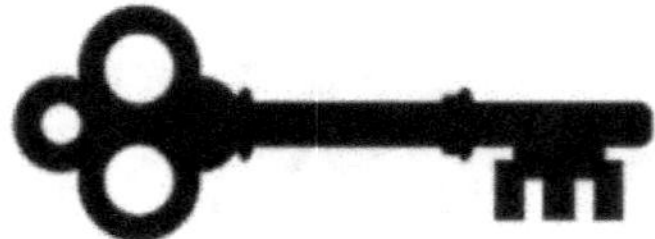

We have arrived at the big secret of LWBE

You must focus all your initial efforts on this basic rule. What you have to do to reach your ideal weight is:

TO CHEW

To chew food until it became almost liquid. As the famous Franciscan friar William of Ockham:

*" The easiest description between equal factors
has to be preferred "*

Among all diets that say everything and the opposite of everything, the best way is to start from the easiest and natural thing to do: To chew our food.

How many slaps in our head have we gotten from our grandparents telling us to Chew!

They were right; they were still living in a human-scale world! This simple attitude means to start to digest food in the mouth and to prepare it for the future digestive processes, in the best way possible. Our body uses a lot of energies for each meal to nourish itself, with each bite; we relieve the digestive energy used during consumption. Consequently, we will have more energy for the other functions, above all brain work. On the contrary, when food reaches our stomach almost still solid, a sense of satiety will arrive very late, because, first pieces must be melted to get nourishment and then to communicate to our brain that we are full. In this way, we will eat more than necessary, and to digest, we will need more energy. To compensate for this effort, the body needs more food and consequently, it assimilates it much more. Now we are inside the vicious circle: I eat by consuming food than I digest badly and I need more energy to absorb it, so I ate more food to consuming it and... the process starts again. After a few years, I became fat without realizing the reasons.

Furthermore, after a while, you will get used to eating unusually, swallowing in greedy and irrationally way, so often, that it becomes a serious medical compulsive problem. Lets' add sedentary life, junk food, stress, and different exaggerations, such as sweets and alcohol and game over.

Think again, everything started from not chewing well the pieces of food that arrives almost intact in our stomach. Sense of satiety needs much more time to communicate to the brain that we are full.

So in these 20 minutes, we ate much more food. Is it so easy? It is enough to start to chew? Yes, it's so easy.

When we introduce foods in our mouth, it is chewed, and it melts together with saliva, and it takes the name of " Bolus." Saliva contains amylase and ptyalin; they are very powerful enzymes that begin to decompose the big starch molecules in more simple sugar molecules. These finally give us the sense of satiety. To end this process, it was estimated to take at least one minute, yes, you read that right one minute to grind and knead bolus, to prepare it for the next step to be swallowed and to reach the stomach. At this point, bolus becomes a semi-liquid mass, named chimo, and it's ready to be digested. This operation takes from one to five hours, according to the bolus and food consistency. After that, chyme is absorbed by the small intestine, named scientifically, duodenum. In this place, the digestion of chyme is completed in the presence of pancreatic juice and bile. The first one contains enzymes that digest proteins by breaking them up in amino acids, by separating carbohydrates in simple sugars and finally by melting fats in fatty acids and glycerol.

Bile is produced by the liver and contains bile salts; this substance emulsifies fats so that you can digest them easily. After a few hours, the absorbed substances now reach the large intestine, and they stay there often for some days. Here, water proteins and mineral salts are absorbed. Here, because of the presence of many useful bacteria (intestinal bacterial flora) that eat the remained substances, it leads to the production of very important vitamins such as B1, B2, and K.

It's a very complicated process. The energy required is very much. If you start on the wrong foot, you create a chain reaction that compromises all digestive processes.

On the contrary, to chew food reduces a lot of this severe danger because bolus arrives at the stomach, ready to become chyme in a relatively short time. If you change this basic factor, you will find yourself completely out of physical fitness with consequent results. Furthermore, not chewed or swallowed food cause an important fermentation that creates a huge production of gases so that the volume of the stomach increases by inflating it. When we eat, the sense of satiety loses itself in the widen and flan three layers of stomach muscles.

The food then has a problem getting in touch with the stomach walls to be transformed and to give a sense of satiety, and we'll continue to eat endlessly. Then gases go down to duodenum and large intestine by filling up all digestive systems and becoming a source of aerophagia. Let's try to control people around us, how many times do they chew their food. I bet that the majority reaches at least 6/10 bites apiece; rather, I'll say that nobody exceeds this number. There are exceptions. Take into consideration one person that looks like you and tries to count: you'll be amazed.

The best doctors in the world are:

DOCTOR FOOD
DOCTOR QUIET
DOCTOR JOY

Chapter 4

LEARN QUICKLY AND EASILY HOW TO PRACTICE THE SECRET

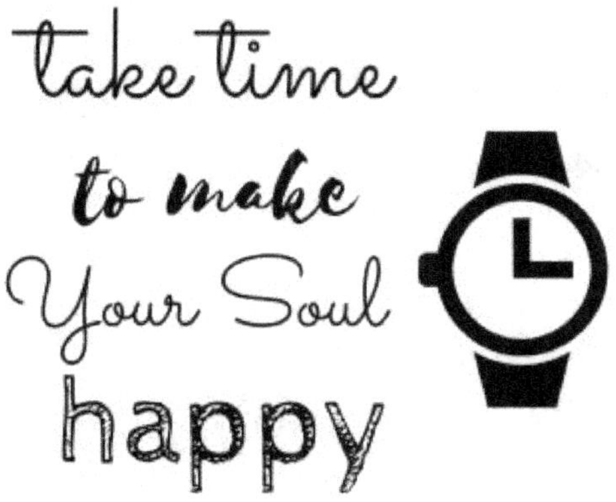

At the very beginning, it seems very difficult to teach your body to change such a rooted attitude for many years. To take time to eat by chewing food, it will be nice and tasty.

You'll realize that food will be much better, and you'll always taste new and tempting flavors. You'll be full much faster, you'll always need smaller rations of food that limit the intake of fats and belly. The more you'll increase the ability to chew, the more you'll feel happy, and your weight will start to decrease. Time to reach ideal weight is different from person to person, but what is important is that this alimentary diet benefit will be so high that you will forget to control how much weight you lose. Other real benefits include serenity energy, happiness, concentration, and more trust in you. Pay attention, I repeat to this very important concept: to chew is an action that needs time. It's useless to stress oneself by counting bites of lunch or dinner until it becomes a nightmare. To chew means to relax by enjoying food, the deep flavors, and aromas.

You'll feel that the more you chew, the more you produce saliva that changes food to bolus and make it paradisiac. So make your peace with this, the goal is to return to ideal weight and to find happiness again. The road is to learn to chew and to observe the other rules of LWBE. To do that, you must face the problem with humility without stressing competitions and without counting bites" and without fierce commitment. Let's start to chew slowly, with a curiosity of a child, and you'll get full success.

The method is foolproof. How can we get used to chewing?

The first rule is very important: you can get all with patience. Start it very slowly, and then increase it. No rush. At the very beginning, leave the scale under your bed, further, we'll start to be friends with it, with due caution. When you eat, learn to relax and to breathe. A very useful suggestion is to lay the fork among morsels of food. Relax in your chair, look around, and enjoy the food that is transforming itself in bolus and it becomes sweet and enjoyable. We lose a lot of flavors if we swallow all at once. The first time, start with 10/15 bites and day by day increase them sweetly. After two weeks, it will be natural; you'll reach the optimal number without even noticing it.

At the end of this chapter, you'll find a program to set up the first month. To train your muscles used to chew, another good suggestion is to chew chewing gum. Classic Modern Chewing gum that conquered the world. It was invented by William sample in the year 1969. Chicle, as it was called by Maya, has a good flavor and trains our mouth to chew constantly and without effort. Furthermore, if it is sugar-free, it can prevent tooth decay. Anyway, what is important is to chew slowly to enjoy food and to take delight in this new lifestyle you're learning.

Only in this way, will you get its benefits, and all the profits that come with it. Smell and watch what you're eating. Smell it until it becomes mouth-watering. Eating is an essential activity for our bodies. Psychologically, to eat satisfies the fundamental needs of primitive man that is still present within us. The basis of his life was to eat, to procreate, and to defend himself from dangers.

Row meat and the quite of caves, shore allowed him to have all possible time to chew and enjoy the hardly conquered food. Often the primitive man is represented as a kind of aggressive and devouring animal with a club. Studies say the contrary: the hunter used to live in places that were populated with many prey, and it was almost easy to feed himself. There were few dangerous predators around, spaces were huge and the man knew exactly how to defend himself, the rare times when he met dangerous animals. We can easily understand that his life was quiet and peaceful. He uses to eat easily. Studies about this, found that, his teeth were made exactly to chew food many times before swallowing.

Families of gorillas and chimpanzees that live in the forest are the clearest proof to confirm how our ancestors used to live. They spend the majority of their life in herds where they live peacefully and quietly. They eat slowly chewing different types of fruits and delights the forest gives them. They always move and the word stress is unknown. They feel it only when herd chief must protect their territory and their females from unwanted intruders; above all, when they reproduce themselves. It concerns short straights among muscled males full of testosterone. It happens 2/3 times a year. LWBE tries to teach us to feed ourselves in the natural and best way possible, as it has been from time immemorial. We could say that it deletes the modern consumerist culture, and brings us back to consider food as a "holy" friend, from which it depends on our life. After some time, while you are practicing this main rule, you will know the moment to swallow food from the consistency of the morsel. Flavors are mixed and all tastes of new, tasting, and inviting. Your body will almost force you to swallow bites; such contentment will let you discover that what you have in your dish is always a little bit more than required. This happens because bolus has reached your stomach has become a sugary food, and it's absorbed immediately, giving you that sense of satiety. Have you ever tried to eat 2 candies or 2 little spoons of sugar before eating? The feeling of satiety will arrive fast before the usual, and you would quietly stop to eat. As soon as you approach the LWBE, you will start to change the measures of your portions, which by now can be decreased. They won't cause any deprivation on your daily requirements. You'll see that portions of your dishes will be considerably reduced, but flavor satisfaction and satiety will increase out of proportion. This is the secret, and this is what we will do.

Now, we will create a list to define precisely when and how to invest time to make LWBE become a daily attitude. At the moment, we will layout the secret only, and then we will integrate it with other rules.

1) **<u>First step</u>**: how many bites do you give to your meal, the first week independently from whatever bites you will give, bring them to 10.

2) **<u>The second week</u>** increase them to 15 steadily and preferring fish and vegetable

3) **<u>The third week</u>** 20 bites a meal and train yourself to eat quietly without any rush by preferring fruits, sweet, and white meats.

4) **<u>The fourth week</u>** chew 25 times and eat fruits, vegetables, fish, and red meats.

5) **<u>At the end of the month</u>**, let your morsel become liquid and tasty.

You should consider that during prolonged chewing, part of the food will be swallowed accidentally.

These are bites of food ready to become bolus and are swallowed because they are ready for the stomach. There are some basic rules to respect, and further we will study them in deep.

At the moment, let's learn that carbohydrates such as Pasta, bread, cereal, and sugars are worse partners of proteins during digestion. Proteins belong to the animal world, and some kinds of plants such as soy belong to the vegetable world. If you eat a nice dish of pasta and the second entry of meat, it means that you are choking your stomach. Avoid it.

This first-month work on chewing and on purify your bad alimentary attitudes such as avoiding mixed foods. When you have your lunch or dinner, choose carbohydrates and vegetables or on the contrary proteins and vegetables, obviously a cake at the end is more good than bad.

"Nothing else than an evolution toward an intelligent or vegetarian diet will ensure a possibility of survival on the earth"

Albert Einstein

Chapter 5

HOW TO TREAT YOUR MEALTIME

It is very important to make your mealtime as a "holy" time, dedicated only to the joy of eating and nothing else.

Concentrate, try to remove all external bothers, and you will see that, day by day, it will be relatively easy to focus on what is in front of you and that you are about to enjoy. Taste all smells and flavors that born in your mouth, and that increase second after second. It does not matter if you are in a five-star restaurant or the bar under your office: use this secret. Eating is always an action that deserves devotion because it's very important for our physical and mental life; and LWBE tries to teach exactly this: Give priority to food and to the new way to eat, this will allow you to get back to that ideal weight. When you are at the table, talk about food and its goodness. Concentrate all your senses on what you are doing. Taste and smell have an important role, both of them invites us to a major enjoyment of eating.

To see what you eat has great importance too. The preparation and serving of food, named "flattening," has become one of the most important sectors of the high-level cuisine.

 It's a real art that shows the dish in the way to be admired and enjoyed by the eyes, by preparing us to its delicious taste which was promised us by the beauty of its composition.

To admire what you are eating creates desire, and helps to identify food taste.

To see freshly baked crisping bread, smelling for its freshness, stimulates all our senses in unison.

It creates that sweaty sensation of mouth-watering that increases our proportion and the desire to eat. Then, if you taste it by chewing it many times, its flavor becomes paradisiac. It's important to live our food in this way; otherwise, you run the risk of losing the main goal, to eat in the best way, without exceeding in quantity. While you are at the table, talking about something else will be less pleasant this moment, above all in the presence of stressing or inappropriate arguments.

Another important suggestion is to chew with a close mouth. This, besides being an education rule that many people have forgotten, permits you to enjoy food in the right way without interruptions or distractions. To chew with our mouths closed doubles the production of saliva with consequent derivative benefits. If you have dinner with friends, take part with joy to that cheerful moment with them and, at the same time, try to give significance to your chewing; maybe listening to them a little bit more and talking only when your piece of food or your dish is finished.

These are simple suggestions that will help you, initially, and then with the habit everything will be natural. The LWBE, with its secret and its corollary advice, establish an alimentary system that brings our body to consume only the quantity of food it needs, according to the requirements of its activity.

We reach the ideal weight because, many calories we eat are in excess; if we stop the thoughtless contribution of food to which we are used to, our body will start to consume the reserve of fat to reach a weight that is proportioned to our physique. The actions that we do together with the secret help this process. Steady Gym, good hydration, the choice of healthy food, specific supplements, and other suggestions you will find in this book will lead you to live healthily.

The system that regulates the appetite is complex, and even scientists still try to learn all the secrets. Some British experts reveal the surprising secrets about the first primary instinct of hunger necessary to survival. The sense of repletion is given by ingested food and by its nutrients above all sugars. Cells of gastrointestinal tract rule the assumed nutrients and, according to them, produce satiety hormones. We say that, we need almost 20 minutes before the stomach starts to feel full and to send to our brain that wonderful sense of satiety.

After a few minutes, we can listen to our sense of satiety, and act accordingly.

If we start to feel full, we can take into consideration that wise Japanese proverb that says:

" *stand up from the table when your belly is almost full* "

You need some willpower to stop our desire to continue to eat, but exercise shows that in one month, you see the first important results. You see food for what it is. You'll appreciate, and respect it. You will come back to be master of eating under all points of view so that naturally, you'll lose weight.

"A meal without wine is almost a day without sun"

Anthelme Brillat Savarin

Chapter 6

THE FOUR ESSENTIAL NUTRITIONAL SUPPLEMENTS FOR GUARANTEED RESULTS

As far as the matter of alimentary supplements is concerned, to adopt together with LWBE we can say that you can do totally without them, even if it is a smart action. It creates a base of all principal substances. This helps to avoid finding ourselves with a deficiency of some minerals, vitamin, or indispensable items for our metabolism, which can lead to health complications. You have to consider that in our society all the food sector is in the hands of multinationals and we know precisely how they think. Try to eat your grandfather's tomatoes from his vegetable garden rather than that one of supermarket close to your house. We will talk about it specifically further on.

Now, let's get back on track.

When you run, you sweat, and you need water. During summer months, above all, you can use some mineral salts, or in their place you can add vegetables and fresh fruit in your meals. Water will keep heat away and will help you to bear with the long, muggy months.

Vitamins have a little special chapter aside. In a varied and balanced diet, plenty of vitamins and mineral salts are enough for the energy requirement of everybody.

Sometimes we live stressful and inhuman life. I suggest you try, at least two times a year, any multivitamin treatment, to have s more weapons to guarantee victory on every daily battle that involves us, maybe in the change of season or after a disease. I suggest you also take two vitamins that I consider fundamental: Vitamin C and vitamin B. Sure they will be present optimally in the basic supplement, but some time to double the amount, it is good and right. I copy down from Wikipedia and the internet what these two vitamins represent in our body.

VITAMIN C

It's important for the connected function of the immune system and the collagen synthesis of the body. The collagen strengthens blood vessels, skin, mussels, and bones. To produce collagen, one needs vitamin C. A continuous supply must synthesize it, Vitamin C has a vital role in all reactions of oxide reduction, which are catalyzed by oxygenizes. It carries out an antihistamine action. Vitamin C or ascorbic acid is widely spread in plants; a very important reserve finds itself in the adrenal glands, in the times of more tension this reserve decreases considerably. This vitamin prevents capillary bleeding, it is also a powerful antioxidant, blocks body aging, and the destructive action of free radicals, and it balances vitamin E levels. This has the same importance of vitamin C for the body.

Vitamin C plays a fundamental role also for the harmonic development of the body and tissue repair. It's important to stimulate wound healing.

As far as the brain, Vitamin C is charged to create the neurotransmitter named norepinephrine that helps to control the use of substances contained in the blood, particularly of glucose.

Daily requirements are around 200 mg (milligrams). Sources of Vitamin C are fruits and fresh vegetables such as guava and especially citrus fruits such as lemons, oranges, and grapefruits; other alimentary sources among vegetables are berries, honey melon, watermelon, kiwi, peppers asparagus, turnip tops, broccoli, cabbages and cabbages flower, potatoes, spinach, and tomatoes.

The maximum amount of vitamin in one food item is in the grape juice, it's cheap and convenient at the same time. Vitamin C is very fleeting, it is destroyed by cooking, by conservation, and by the exposition to light and air; that is why it is important to eat fresh food.

The fresher and less cooked they are, the more the quantity of Vitamin. Among the preferred cooking techniques we have, microwave oven, stem, and quick frying.

Kiwi has a major quantity of C vitamin imagine that in 6 kiwis, we'll find 500 mg of the vitamin.

Supplements broadly cover the needs and give a good stock of vitamins to our body to be used in the hardest periods at its leisure.

VITAMIN B

It has many useful properties for the human body. It plays an essential role in the functioning of the nervous system and the muscle tone of the gastrointestinal area. They are also important for the hairs, skin, scalp, as well as mouth, eyes, and liver. They convert carbohydrates to glucose that is used to produce energy in the body. They are fundamental for lipid and protein metabolism. Vitamins B have many functions, all different and essential for the human body; their provision with diet should be constantly adequate; even if they are molecules mostly stored in the liver, their assumption must respect: first, the recommended reactions and second also individual necessities. There are many kinds of vitamin B, and I suggest taking a look on the Internet to deepen the topic. Just because they are many, they find themselves in many different items of food, and have different functions; we run the risk of having a lack of one of these.

Supplements guarantee we always the right quantity at any given time. If we assume Vitamins C and B together with omega 3 that is found in fish oil capsules and the water daily, they help very much. The majority of times, they make a difference and give us an extra gear in our life, and it is always welcome.

Think about the two Nobel prize winners, one is Dr. Louis Arraign, they discovered a shocking truth; their laboratories found and informed different health departments that, in this world, the main causes of death are due to what we eat to a lesser extent and for the vast majority to what our body lacks.

We are talking about: ischemic heart disease, cardiovascular diseases, cerebrovascular diseases, malignant tumors, depressions, and dementia Alzheimer's. Let's imagine everyone whose breakfast is Coffee and Muffin: this is a wonderful pair that gives you the right charge for the morning. The reality is that most enjoy them day by day, month by month; their diet is based on carbohydrates such as pasta, sugar, animal proteins, heavy seasonings, few vegetables and fruits, and all kinds of food and beverages. After 50 years, how do you think their body and above all their psyche will be? How do they feed their brain? In this century, depression is in the first place among the terrible deficiencies that afflict all of us.

In the pharmacies, the most sold drug is paracetamol, then antidepressants, anxiolytics, tranquilizers, and so on. If you miss something for decades sooner or later, something is going to break. Basic supplement compensates almost totally these deficiencies; it's a great consolation to be protected for all these.

I forgot... It costs as a coffee.

"Sometimes it's difficult to make the right decision between remorses of conscience or hunger bites"

Totò

From The Italian Movie: "The Gang of Criminals"

Chapter 7

HOW TO OVERCOME HUNGER WITHOUT COMMITMENT AND SUFFERING

Slow Down

In this initial step of our journey, it's normal to feel hunger, because we are changing our alimentary attitude from a model to another. What do we do when it attacks us?.

First, we must immediately reduce the working rhythm of our body. If you are walking and you feel hungry, slow down or sit down for a while. If you are in the office, stop your work for a while and breathe. Give your body time to solve this little problem. Our body knows hunger very well and at that moment it must answer to a particular sensation of need, and it must do it together with you in the best way. Once the situation is under control, start to work in steps.

First, drink water, which is our lifeblood, our nectar. In this way, we taste if hunger is real hunger or only thirst.

Is it weird?

The majority of times, our body begs water after many years of bad attitudes and involuntary dehydration.

Doctor Fereydoon Batmanghelidj (difficult surname to pronounce) that we 'll know better in next the chapters says: our body implores water in all possible ways until it feeds that hunger or water.

When hunger makes us feel its bites, we must fight it back by drinking 2 glasses of water at the distance of a couple of minutes, and then let's see. If the situation gets better, you did the right move, your body was only thirsty. On the contrary, if hunger stays, then you will go to the second step called "B plan." Usually, after we drink, the need to eat is alleviated, and we need just a little bit of well-chewed food. Choose fruits or herb teas with whole wheat food. You can also eat a brioche or biscuits what is important is to chew them very well, and they should be "little worked" such as those of industrial begs. A glass of water with a little bit of basic supplement is also advisable or the classic homemade snack, and this is better.

Hunger is only a healthy request for food from the body, and it is easily manageable and controllable. As far as snacks are concerned, try to avoid junk food or super sweetened beverages. They help you at the moment, but they are chemically planned to let you feel more hungry and thirsty than you were before. Sometimes if you feel strong and competitive wait for 20 minutes and hunger will disappear

As if by magic. Try to resist for some minutes, and it will go away. To know that our worse enemy depends on our will, it is a great deliverance! The merciless dictator that wanted all is gone. Stop with the food food food.

After a while, the desire to eat passes, and the more experience you will get with it, the stronger you will be. It is our body's reaction that takes energy from us and it is exactly what we need to use what we have in excess.

So wait for a while and resist. Since I live with this alimentary style, I can say that a few times I felt hunger, I'll say rarely. Another benefit you will have from LWBE is to go to the restaurant. A delicious fish with many vegetables and sweets will be enough for you to feel like you are in paradise. You will be able to live with fewer quantities of food, and consequently, you will pay less, really less, and you will be happy. At home, your food shopping will last twice as long if you cook by yourself, you will save, and it will be substantial. You will appreciate this aspect during the time because it's always a pleasure to have some more money in the pocket. Allow me to make a joke: you will become slim and rich!.

Obviously, as in all problems, there is always the flip side. You will save from aside, but you will spend more in another. Oh yes, months of shopping are waiting for you to buy ever smaller size dresses. Soon you must change your entire wardrobe. Prepare yourself for this future because it will happen. At the very beginning, normally, you lose a size within 4/6 months. After that time dresses slowly will be larger, but you will discover the joy to wear that pair of jeans again in the wardrobe for many years that you loved. Each time you saw them they made you say: you put on weight, do something!

Monthly you will often see your tailor and your preferred dresses shop. They will be happy, but you will be happier. The most exciting expense will be a bath suite, smaller size, and your body always more beautiful. What I wrote till now will seem like an unattainable dream, but you will change your mind!

It will happen, it will really happen.

"If there is magic in this planet it is contained in water"

Loren Eiseley

Chapter 8

YOUR GREATEST ALLY AND HOW TO TAKE ADVANTAGE OF IT DURING THE FIRST MONTH

Our body is composed of 80% water. A little bit more in children and a little less in the old people. Water is so essential for us that without food we can survive for a month on, on the contrary, without water we fly to paradise after few days, for few days I mean those that you can count on the finger of your hands.

Water is the place where all processes occur and permit cells to reproduce and keep themselves alive. She is the main actress of all body functions.

All chemical and organic processes can exist only with their presence. It is the principal part of all human beings. The man-body fluids that are constituted principally by water are Cerebrospinal fluid 99%, Bone marrow fluid 99%, and blood plasma 85%. Water plays an important role in all transportation of nutrients to all body districts, furthermore for the elimination and excretion of dossers throughout urine. Another important water function is the regulation of body temperature, the balance of salt concentration; it takes part in digestion, helping both intestinal transit, and the absorption of nutrients. For all those reasons, water must be present in high quantity in human nutrition, it is classified as an essential macronutrient. Plenty of water means to live in mountain fresh, alive, a luxuriant little lake with a river that flows in bringing nourishment and another one that flows out taking away with him all impurities and debris, by living clean in a livable place. Lake turns quickly into a smelly, putrid lifeless pond populated only by frogs and mosquitoes, without this source. This easy and simple example gives us an idea about how our life could be without it!

To distract means to put in crisis all vital body functions and those of the brain, you feel confused weak and at risk of life. For many years we drink beverages that can replace water, but in reality, they stimulate the need for it. All ads communication tries to confuse us by exposing us to useless and toxic foods.

The majority of us stop drinking "holy" water (holy in the real sense of words) and settle for useless surrogates for the ideal hydration. Unfortunately, it concerns all young people. Imagine being thirsty, really thirsty; your body starts to ask you for water to drink. It's driven from a physical need, and it generates the desire to drink so that we start to look for something to drink; sure to be right, we pull the tab and drink a couple of glasses of a black beverage that is full of sugar, phosphoric acid, caffeine, and much dioxide and a little bit of water just enough. It's colored black because of caramel that, in reality, is sugar melted at 137°. It also contains mysterious flavors, so-called natural flavors. For decades everyone wonders what they could be, but they know perfectly that they are secretly kept inside a safe, its door is 1 meter thick, so nobody will know what they are above all if these natural flavors are toxic or wholesome for our health.

Now, this wonderful beverage that you have just drunk is created studied and tested in all possible ways only to let it give us temporary refreshment, and after less than one hour you will be thirsty again. The consumption of these kinds of beverages is around 800 million cans daily.

What is more ridiculous is that these beverages don't contain any nutrients suitable to quench thirst and to moisturize. Ask yourself a question: is it normal?

Companies bombard us with misleading messages that bring us to consume chemical liquid.

Water is irreplaceable, water is the source of life. All diets in the world have the same fundamental rule: to drink at least 1 or 2 liters of water each day. This rule has to be taken very seriously.

Now that we have cleared its importance, let 's start to hydrate ourselves properly. To get used to the optimal water level that is our daily body requirements, we need almost a month to hydrate, to get to the last cell we need 2 months. This overlaps perfectly with the initial suggestion: to change attitude we need almost 30 days. Start with one, two glasses per day, and remove all trash drinks you got used to during the years. You can also alternate with tea, herb teas, and other beverages composed only of water and natural flavors in the real sense of words.

For the first month, try to drink water even if you are not thirsty because our body needs help to come back to healthy attitudes. After a month, you'll reach your balance, suitable to satisfy daily support of water and you'll get used to drinking regularly.

You'll learn to be another person, I assure it. You'll be in front of the mirror, and you will see a new light inside you. Your mind will be brighter, your vital functions will work at 100%.

Ulcers headache, mussels pains will fade away.

How many people I saw to solve their big problem of chronic constipation in a couple of months.

A couple of liters of water is around 7/8 glasses daily that, together with other sources of supply, will satisfy our total needs. It's an easy goal to reach, and the benefit will be so big that you'll be happy, really happy. Furthermore, water increases spittle helping the production of the bolus in the mouth; this will be turned faster than usual, and it will be more digestible and tasty, every food road will benefit. Water is really important for all functions, digestion inclusive. Revealing signs of good hydration are: transparent urine and always a happy mood.

Let's see now the kind of water to drink.

Personal taste is fundamental. The main thing to do is to choose our preferred water.

Its health features depend on its source of origin and mineral salts that water carries along its underground way through rocks before it gushes to the surface. According to the kinds of dissolved minerals which are indicated as fixed residue, it means the number of deposited minerals of a liter evaporated water at 180°, mineral waters are classified as:

- <u>Minimally mineralized waters</u>:

They have mineral salts less than 50 milligrams per liter. They are "light waters" because they are poor of mineral salts they help diuresis and facilitate the expulsion of small kidney stones.

- <u>Low mineral waters</u>:

They contain a little bit more than 500 milligrams per liter because they have few mineral salts.

They are excellent table waters that you can drink daily. They perform a diuretic action, and they contain a few sodiums.

- <u>Mineral waters</u>

Fixed residue fluctuates between 500 and 1000 milligrams per liter. They contain a substantial quantity of mineral salts, and for that, you should drink them in limited quantity, maximum of one liter a day by alternating them with low mineral waters

Some mineral waters fixed residue is more than 1500 milligrams per liter. They are very rich in salts, for that reason, you should drink them only for healing goals and under medical suggestion. You can buy them both in the pharmacies and supermarkets.

Frankly speaking, I believe that water from your home tap is good enough, but if you can't stand its flavor, you can buy water in bottles. I suggest you give priority to water brands that have their sources not far from where you live to control prices. Near you, it means fewer trucks that move, less pollution, and lower prices. At the very end, you will get used to water flavor soon, and after some weeks, it will have a good taste. A good attitude is always to have a bottle of water handy.

When you drink, be careful to have the right quantity of water and wait for some minutes before drinking again, possibly the same quantity. This way, it will be easier to attain the famous 2 liters a day. If you think that you will frequently visit the restroom, you will be surprised: your body will adjust fast to this cure that we are proposing. The body keeps water as much it can, it will assimilate it in the best possible ways. The result will be that you will go to the bathroom the same number of times, but you will lose more quantity of liquid and toxins.

About this topic, I suggest you read a very interesting book, " Your Body's Many Cries for Water " written by doctor Fereydoon Batmanghelidj.

This Iranian doctor wrote many texts about the dehydration of the human body and about the serious problems it may cause. In the 80s, after the coup d'etat in Iran, during his imprisonment, he got to these conclusions. At that time, Fereydoon Batmanghelidj, thanks to his medical background, was saved from death because he was encharged as a doctor to take care of prisoners. However, prisoners were abandoned to their fate from jailers to die or to be executed.

Stress was very high, and he couldn't work as a doctor. The situation was dramatic, and so he treated ulcers and the most severe problems of prisoners with the only medicine he had available: water and the prisoners got better!

The major benefits were in the dysfunction of the digestive system and the treatment of psychic problems. In 1982 he was set free from prison, so doctor Fereydoon Batmanghelidj went to the United States of America, and he established "the foundation of simplified medicine" that is still studied today and spreads his revolutionary discover: lack of water as a simple cause of many diseases. This disclosure changed my life literally. To drink water means letting our body in a perfectly fresh and racy environment. There are also excellent healthy beverages such as wine, beer, milk, fruit juices, and supplements. You can drink all of them, and they are all allowed, however, drink them mildly because the real nectar is always water.

    Caffeine and alcohol dehydrate us very much, and if they are assumed, it's better to drink more than the recommended 2 liters of water per day.

PAY ATTENTION to water: should be kept far away during meals, it should be taken 1 hour before and 12 hours later. This stops the gastric juices from eating during digestion.

ONCE SAID THAT: PROSIT!

SUMMARY:

THE ACTIONS TO MAKE THIS FIRST MONTH :

- **The first week**: half a liter of water integrating with a little bit of tea.

- **The second week**: drink 5 glasses of water daily and relaxing herb tea in the evening

- **The third week**: 7 glasses of water and tea or herb teas depending on the quantity you want.

- **The fourth week**: 10 water glasses, tea herb teas at your pleasure

From the end of the month on, drink 8 glasses of water, teas, herb teas, and at maximum coffee, beer, and mildly alcoholic drinks.

Remember :

Drink water away from principal meals.

"Sushi it's much more than to put fish in the rice: sushi is a kind of art "

Jiro Ono

Chapter 9

ONE OF THE MOST IMPORTANT ESSENTIAL FOODS

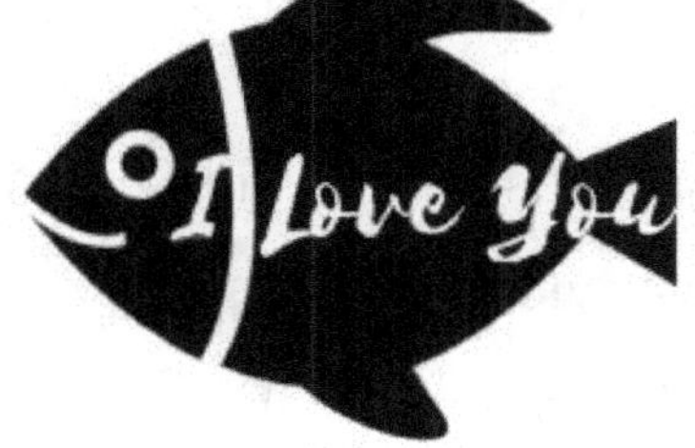

In this section, we will talk deeply, and learn how to get the attitude to eating very important food for our body and life: fish. The word fish is used to consider all that comes from water; in reality, fish, according to science, indicates all water vertebrates with gills and fins.

Their body structure differentiates them from mollusks and shellfish, and it's always an important food landmark. It has great nutritional qualities because it brings high biological value proteins, unsaturated fatty acids (among them Omega 3), minerals, salts such as phosphorus, iodine, selenium, and Vitamins A, D, and B. The reduced quantity of connective tissue in the fish, makes it very digestible.

Nowadays, unfortunately, it is not so present in our diet because it's difficult to find and cook.

You should integrate fish into your diet. Our grandmother gave us a nasty cod oil to drink, and she was right!

At that time, it was almost impossible to find it except along the sea coasts, it was not well known and, however, rarely eaten. Nowadays, you can buy it all over, but the little knowledge of consumers and the fear that it's not all that fresh means it rarely on our tables. In our frantic society, there is no time to clean and cook it.

In the end, we hate to wash stinking dishes. Classic fish in cans it is very far from our need. Preservatives, additives, and flavors contained inside denature completely its organoleptic properties, so that, it smells colorful but poorly nutritious.

Here is a little fish range that mother nature presents us so that you will have clearer ideas when you choose.

Science classifies different kinds of fishes according to different standards.

From a biological point of view, they distinguish in:

Sea fish: they live offshore, and are the major part of all living species.

Freshwater fish: they live in rivers and lakes, and they are in small quantities.

Mixed water fish: they live in places where there is a mixture of two kinds of water, such as: in the river mouths and coastal lagoons. Some fishes migrate spending part of their life in freshwaters and the other part in salted waters.

Fishes can be categorized according to nutritional characteristics and particularly according to the number of fats.

Lean fish are characterized by 3% of fat, such as sole sea bream, turbot fish, cod, pike, dogfish, and grouper.

Half fat fish: 3-9% of fats and they are: anchovy, carp, tuna fish, trout, swordfish, sardine, mullet, bream

Fat fish contain more than 9% of fats such as eel, mackerel, salmon.

This list has to be taken with attention because fat quantity changes very much; it depends on the age and the biological cycle.

As far as their meat storage is concerned, we will talk about:

Fresh fish that is not frozen. It must have firm consistency, compacted meat, red gills, and shiny scales. It must have a live eye, a nice and not very intense flavor. Fresh fish must be conserved in the coolest place of the fridge, and it must be consumed within 24 hours of purchase.

Frozen fish

It's treated with a method that brings the central part of the product to -18°. Outside it is covered in ice, and it is named icing. It preservers fish from oxidation. About storage, you must follow the rules indicated on the package.

Deep frozen fish

All its parts are frozen at a temperature of -18° in a little time. Also, in this case, it is undergoes icing treatment. Indications for storage must be showed in the package.

If the fish is correctly frozen, it keeps all of its organoleptic properties, and it is a good alternative to the fresh product.

Preserved fish

It is made with different kinds of techniques that in different ways change its nutritional qualities.

The most well-known methods are:

-salting

It can be done dry or stewed salting. It's used for sardines, mackerels, and anchovies.

-drying

It could be natural at air exposition or artificial, it's used for lean fishes.

-smoking

fish is salted, dried, and then smoked (with smoke coming from burning wood).

It is used on salmon, sardine, cod, mackerel, and herrings.

Canning

After washing, cooking, and drying fish, it's placed in oil or a saline solution. It's used for tuna fish, sardines, anchovies, and mackerel.

Clams are a separate category.
These animals have a flabby body that gives them the name.
They are divided into three big categories:

CEPHALOPODS

They do not have a shell or have it inside their body: they are squids, octopus cuttlefish, baby octopus.

GASTROPODS

They are made of one valve only. They are limpets, murici fish, sea and earth snail, abalone.

LAMELLIBRANCH

They have two valves, shell, and they are MITILI CLAMS, OYSTERS, SEA TRUFFLES, TELLINS, SEA DATES BEAMS.

Fresh or frozen mollusks caught or famed are easily found in the market.

Nowadays, there are fixed rules as far as fishing breeding, sales, and transportation are concerned.

Nutritionally speaking, mollusks have a good quantity of proteins, polyunsaturated fatty acids, and mineral salts. Among them, sodium, potassium, calcium, iron, iodine, and vitamins A and B.

Then we find the shellfish category. They have an external hard articulated body.

There are many species, but the most well known in the food field are lobster, crayfish, crabs, escape, and mantis shrimps. You can find both fresh and frozen ones. But you should pay attention to the dark spots on the shell that appear progressively over time, they should be few, and the smell should be nice.

Shellfish contain proteins in reasonable quantity; they have a large portion of cholesterol, vitamins B, mineral salts such as iodine, phosphorus, sodium, and potassium. I suggest you take them together with a basic supplement, fish oil, omega 3 capsules. They work very well when they give you lucid and good. They are simply practical and cheap. They cover almost all the body needs, and you will avoid the nasty taste of the grandmothers' beloved cod liver oil.

In the market, you can find many kinds of omega 3 capsules and for all budgets. I tried almost all the brands, and I will say that all of them can be good.

Take them in the right quantity, you'll find it in the package, and after some time, you will decide to take them according to your needs and according to your body's response to the product.

By taking fish oil in this way, you will have a good provision of useful fish substances.

Take into consideration that Fish oil capsules Omega3 are supplements, and they cover almost all your needs. To eat fish twice a week will complete the necessity.

Nowadays, with modern transportation and storage treatments, such as the cutting down of fish products at very low temperature immediately after fishing, all fishes that arrive in shop counters are all fresh and eatable. In supermarkets, packs of lean fish are good, sure you need imagination about seasoning, maybe a good recipe to enhance the flavor.

Since the transportation service is so fast that it arrives at the fish supermarkets of inland cities in time, it also adds to the cost. So keep calm in front of the fish counter! Strict market laws ensure that fresh and healthy products arrive at your tables. Let your preferred fishmonger suggests what you need to buy and how to cook it. There are many easy, tasty recipes to prepare, and when you have time, go to the stove and try to create some excess with this amazing product of nature.

You will see that it is easier than what you think...

For the rest.. there is a dishwasher!

" A nice walk of 5 km is more effective for an unhappy man than all drugs and psychologists in the world "

Paul Dudley White

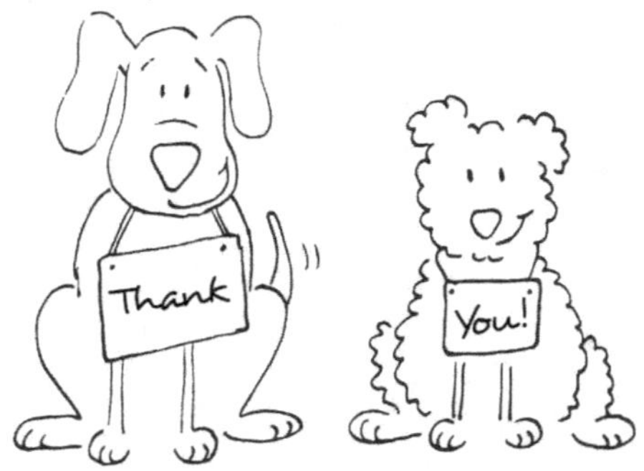

Enjoying this book so far?
I hope that You could take some time to post a quick review
on Amazon!

Chapter 10

HOW TO TAKE BACK CONTROL OF YOUR BODY

While we are continuing on our journey to learn to practice our alimentary diet, we reach this chapter that shows one of the most basic topics about LWBE.

A great philosopher of our times wrote that man is a moving social animal.

Unfortunately, socialization in our current life is deeply changed. We are more alone than 502 years ago. TV Computer and large urban agglomeration created loneliness and all connected diseases. Furthermore, the social moving man has become stationary in industrialized countries.

A normal office clerk spends almost 9.3 hours daily, mostly sitting and physically inactive, time to sleep aside. Even if it is an average data and changes from job to job and from nation to nation, it's always terrifying data. Try to realize it: Practically, we remain inactive for 36 years of our life. This attitude does not suit our hunters, pickers, shepherds, and peasants' body. This life of half immobility brings us to many and severe diseases, among them heart problems, depression, strokes, and diabetes, and naturally obesity with all its consequences. From many statistics, it's clear that in the richest countries, the percentage of people with a sedentary life is around 51%. Half of the people around you spend their time among computers, sofas, cars and office chairs without a little movement.

Sixty years ago, these people were less than 10% of the population. This is a serious problem, and we must get out of it quickly. As we said, researchers discovered that among the most used drugs we find in the first place: anti-flu, psychopharmaceuticals, and guess what? In the third place, we find drugs relative to sedentary: such as muscle pains due to wrong postures, sight deterioration, arthritis diabetes, heart problems, blood circulation, insomnia, and chronic fatigue. Sedentary strongly increases the possibility of falling in more or less severe neurosis conditions. You passively face all stress and painful situations common to everybody, without a healthy and strong body. This kind of pliable behavior causes a lack of problem resolution and, consequently, severe self-esteem and interior peace risks. The only solution to problems related to sedentary is to start to sweat, move the body, and replace sofas and chairs with tracksuit and sneakers. This is a fundamental rule of LWBE! I'll say that this is the third one, the first one is: "Miss water." If you play sports regularly, lucky you, but if you belong to that 80% of people that types on computers, write with a pen in front of a desk daily or you are ground from stressful responsibilities, it's time to make a decision and change your lifestyle. It's time to make the right decision without any fears. We'll start with relaxing and less tiresome exercises. The only goal will be to know the happiness that you feel when you start to move. The first time playing sports will be only to sweat a little bit.

LWBE uses this happiness to let us come back to an ideal weight and give us mental and physical health. Let's see carefully what happens when we start to play sports.

It affects endorphin and serotonin levels, which are released from our body, and it brings us to a good mood. Endorphins are endogenous opiates; in other words, chemical substances of organic nature produced by the brain.

They have analgesic and physiological features similar to those found in morphine and opium but of wider range; furthermore, they are naturally assimilated from the body.

Endorphins can cause such feelings of euphoria and peace, more or less intense, according to the released quantity, such as many alkaloids, which is derived from morphine.

They are produced from the body during sports activity, such as during sex, kisses, falling in love, contact, caresses, a nice massage, and even when you taste cocoa. The release of these substances alleviates pains, which is why they got the name "happiness hormone":

The synthesis of endogenous opiates increases according to body exercise. Even if this is subjective, plasma concentrations raise on average of 500%. This explains clearly that feeling of Euphoria and well being that happens after we played physical activity. You feel a considerable reduction of anxiety and stress from anger. Hunger control is another good consequence, together with a potent analgesic effect caused by a reduced perception of pains.

Think about what we loose in the sedentary weeks we are used to.

Now let's talk about how to face our first steps to start a physical activity. Primarily, it's important that our first goal is only to hit our body and feel that it reacts again to movement. Endorphins will start to work slowly and they'll let you feel that well being of "soul."

I'll give you an example: if you work or live on the 5th floor, say bye-bye to the elevator and walk steps slowly. The second day when you'll be on the second floor, you will call the ambulance! After a month, you will walk all floors taking two steps at a time. You will arrive happily and smiling, and your day will change radically. As the days go on, you will start to go out on foot. Then you will walk all steps of the buildings. The endorphin you will gain from avoiding the elevator will give you that happiness, it will be the boost to better and improve your physical exercises.

There are many ways to work. Some of them are nice too. For example, you close yourself in a room wearing headphones and dance for 20 minutes. Music endorphins and sweat make miracles!

The first days you will think that you are mad, but over time, John Travolta that is inside you will come out, and dancing will be your favorite Sport.

Before talking about gym exercises and strategies to get the most out of it, we should talk a little bit about the knowledge of our essential friend to carry on our new adventure. It is a virtue that should be in the first place of our commitment: Constancy.

In the very beginning, it can scare you, but in reality, it is our best friend. Before starting to move, it is essential to understand that constancy is more important than sweat. It does not matter which sport you play, where you play it, and how much time you spend on it, it will be essential to practice it steadily. If you run for a week, and then you stop, it means nothing. It's better to walk and do it always. The first important training to learn is to be faithful to the established program. You need firmness, strength, and choice and after one month, it will be easy to overcome the effort. It will be your body asking you to move with remarkable benefits. At first, it will be necessary to program some specific training and then follow it the most possible. Walk steps, give up the car, or simply do a little bit of light gym or dance. One of the best movements is to stroll into the green, maybe with a friend, or if you live in a town in cold seasons, buy a tapis Roulant (Treadmill).

You can find them on the internet at an affordable price. Tapis Roulant (Treadmill) is usually kept under our bed, and if you use it steadily, it replaces a walk because it simulates perfectly it. In wintertime, you will appreciate it very much, of course, open-air and a park is the best. It's good enough to have a home gym, on the internet, there are many funny and instructive videos. Among all home sports, the best one is to dance or jump with a rope. I would like to talk a little bit about this simple, almost unknown exerciser. Certainly, each one of us played it when young. In reality, it is a real sports training; with simple exercises, only 20 minutes of it is the same as 40 minutes of jogging, and you burn 350 calories which are the equivalent of:

- 180 grams of cooked chicken

- 1 dish of grilled vegetables

- 1 dish of salad

- 1 dish of brown rice

- 2 oil spoons

- 2 vinegar spoons Not bad at all!

To jump with a rope is a typical aerobic activity, it betters the coordination, increases lung capacity, and cardiac resistance. It is used by boxers and professional sportsmen as well as many show stars because it promises snappy, limb legs, and a marble B side. If you choose to use it as a basic sport together with our alimentary diet, it guarantees excellent results after 4 weeks of practice. Initially, if you have problems coordinating movement, you can start to jump without rope simulating the rotation. On the Internet, you can watch a lot of videos that teach the basic steps to start to jump and to set your training to the best.

Other benefits of rope are low price, it's easy to use, and it is not cumbersome. You can use it all over, open-air, inside a gym during your vacations, and why not during your work break. You'll immediately start to sweet and high heartbeat attack fats at once. There are many other benefits. If you jump ropes while you're listening to your favorite music, this kind of training is similar to a game. As soon as you can control the rotating rope, you will feel a healthy addiction and much happiness. To jump with a rope has a playful pleasure in it, that helps us to continue our training even if we feel lazy, we find many excuses, and we want to sink in our sofa. Music, video, rhythm, and the capacity to coordinate in the gesture of movement, makes our training immediately pleasant and exciting, above all because it is a real cure for our humor and inner balance.

If you can join a gym, you can train yourself easily with a variety of available equipment. At first, it is important that after training the muscles sweetly, then a 20 minutes stretch is essential to prepare your body for rest. Remember that you are there to sweat a little bit, without bodybuilding world championship ambitions. Talk with your trainer and let him show you specific movements to give to your body the right posture. After many years of inactivity, you take the classic tortoise position that is the same one when you sit on the sofa. The back is hunched, the neck falls between the shoulder blades, and the belly comes out out of proportion. This posture causes cervical and dorsal pains, and from an aesthetic point of view, it generates a deformed belly to the outside. We won't talk about the postures caused by smartphones while you are chatting or sending messages. There we reach the height of the tops.

Muscles used to tighten your back from shoulders to buttocks and so it's useless and dangerous to do only exercises for abs and pectorals to be more beautiful. We will bend more seriously, and we will worsen the situation. Besides, to create a month's training scheduled, it's important someone shows you some exercises for your fatty parts. Above all, for all our female friends, it's good to start with specific exercises for legs and buttocks and then move on to other parts of the body. If you can make some plans, you have all my approval.

When you train a specific part, all body benefits from it.

While you are attending a gym, it would be appropriate to make new friends. This helps to be constant, and it distracts from efforts and monotony. If I should suggest some other nice and involving sport, I'll say to you to find out if there are dance halls in your area, where you can do one of the many dances practiced in the world: modern, classic, caraibic or group dances. Alternatively, you can practice some gentle aerobic lesson. Music is a friend of life and endorphins and it promotes friendships and human contact. I believe that Music was invented by God on the seventh day, as an immense gift for our happiness. What can we find that is similar to it? To dance is a way that can illuminate the monotonous people's lives. It gives benefits to emotional, physical, mental, and general health.

Dance is a real art, and it brings unimaginable benefits. To dance is just that ... joy and happiness. It reduces blood pressure prevents cardiovascular diseases, lowers cholesterol level, increases muscle tone, and is socially useful because it helps to find out new friendships. Think about south American dances such as "salsa" or Spanish tango or smooth dance, all of them bring people to have contacts and feel good physically and mentally. Remember the endorphins that emanate from caresses and touch. If you are embarrassed because you are overweight and you don't feel like going to a club nearby to nice slim, attractive toned dancers, you can watch videos on the internet and train yourself, waiting for time to get out from your cocoon and fly like a butterfly to a "vaulting parquet" (dance floor) maybe with friends or girlfriends.

Believe me, music makes miracles!

 As soon as the beautiful season comes, you can indulge yourself with what you love most—strolling, race, horse. You must be steady, this is significant. I'll repeat it a thousand times: be constant.

Repeat it to yourself: **I'm constant** !

In hot months, swimming is the best. It relaxes and trains all muscles perfectly. If you have a swimming pool near your house, take the opportunity and dive into it. A few strokes are enough or stay in the water making slow movements, and the game is done. If the swimming pool also has a sauna or Turkish bath, try to use them. They are soothing and purifying. In sports, the movement allows unavoidably one to come out of oneself and look at oneself. When you are on a bike or in a swimming pool or underweights in your gym, open your mind, forget problems, let yourself go. Try to relax, listen to nice music, or talk with someone about light topics. To look around us creates tranquility and increases happiness and constancy. Life is to go out of ourselves!

Our Thoughts are completely different from others. People see us in different ways, we believe.

When you are training, and you think that others look at you with contempt because you are overweight, 90% of the time, it is wrong. Also, others have more or less the same thoughts about themselves that you have about yourself. We are all in the same boat. Communication helps much, you can start a friendship, and you know: Whoever finds a friend finds a treasure. Cheer up! Throw away your sofa, burn your TV remote control, your body wants to move, it begs you to move.

Talk about sports. You are together with other people that could stay near you and help you. Maybe they were as chubby as you, certainly, they'll understand very well the effort you are making and they can help you in difficult moments. Furthermore, within a team, everybody takes care of his teammate, and so you will feel protected as if within a herd. However, pay attention to the competition.

Do you know that the majority of football injuries happen during the classic matches bachelors versus husbands, where competition is strong, but the body is weak and untrained?

Everyone feels like Maradona, but then different kinds of ligaments and dislocations are the prize of the game, and to heal only one of them, takes three times more when you were young.

Come on, get busy, reborn to a new life.

Believe me, to move is fundamental. It's fun. Many people completely forget the joy of training their bodies. How it's beautiful to sweat and then to drink fresh water. How much happiness you derive in a race and a warm shower, and then when you go to bed to feel tired but satisfied.!

You are creating an alimentary and physical way that involves all your life at 360 °, and it will deeply better every aspect of it.

There is another very important suggestion I would like to give you. When you start to move and to make your diet, periodically, take pictures of yourself when you are naked. It will help you to see your progress stage after stage. You will be amazed to see how fast your LWBE will work. Weight scale also will give you only good news, believe it, be sure of it. You can do it too. Be convinced, be steady.

"Every morning in Africa when the sun rises a gazelle wakes up and knows that it will have to run faster than the lion. Every morning in Africa when the sun rises a lion wakes up and knows that it will have to run faster than the gazelle"

African Saying

Chapter 11

YOUR EASY 10-WEEK WORK PLAN

WEEK 1

1 minute light race alternated with 2 minutes of walking for 9 times (total 27 minutes

WEEK 2

2 minutes of light race alternated with 3 minutes of walking for 6 times (tot. 30 minutes)

WEEK 3

4 minutes of light race alternated with 3 minutes of walking for 5 times (tot. 35 minutes)

at the end of these weeks, you will feel more vital, active and reactive... pay attention anyway do not exaggerate, next weeks will be more beautiful.

WEEK 4

6 minutes of light race alternated with 3 minutes of walking for 5 times (45 minutes)

WEEK 5

10 minutes of light race alternated with 3 minutes of walking for 4 times (tot. 52 minutes)

WEEK 6

15 minutes of light race alternated with 3 minutes of walking for 3 times (tot. 54 minutes)

Now you should start feeling fit. You are beginning to walk a few kilometers. A little more than a month ago you were a sofa sloth, and now you feel more vital and active, you start to better your body too. What do you want more? To continue.

WEEK 7

25 minutes of light race alternated with 3 minutes of walking for 2 times (Tot. 56 minutes)

WEEK 8

40 minutes of light race (first exit) Monday

40 minutes of light race (second exit) Tuesday

(according to your daily plan)

45 minutes of light race (third exit) Friday

WEEK 9

45 minutes of light race (exit 1)

50 Minutes of light race (exit 2)

(according to your daily plan)

50 minutes of light race (exit 3)

WEEK 10

1 hour of light race or 10 kilometers walking (1 exit only)

As far as it concerns walking just replace walking with race.

" To eat is one of four goals of life...nobody knows which are the other three ones "

Chinese saying

Chapter 12

YOUR BEST FOOD COMBINATIONS

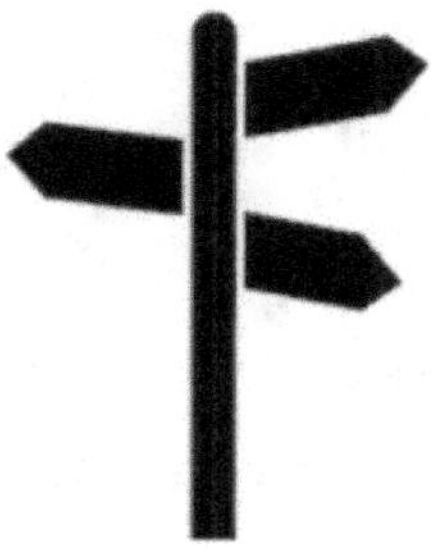

There is a Japanese saying that says:

"Stand up from the table with your belly almost full."

I believe this to be one of the best strategies to live in perfect ideal weight and healthily the longest possible way. It's the same with LWBE . We'll learn to eat a little bit less, but we'll feel more satiated than before. Much more satiated than before.

By practicing the secret LWBE, the body gets used to eating only what it needs to feel satiated, by avoiding accumulations that become fats. You will be able to reach an ideal weight in a few months if you also follow side rules, such as, drinking water, playing sport steadily and eating genuine food, furthermore, you get in a diet that guarantees the joy of life all life long. Well, lets' move to the fundamental question of this chapter: What can you eat? ALL. yes you understood correctly. You can eat everything.

At the very beginning with some forethought, then by time, it will be an attitude. Then when you are better, you will easily handle food and its characteristics by yourself. To chew, let you discover many new flavors. To turn food into bolus gives off fantastic aftertastes that we have completely forgotten while eating voraciously. Fruits and vegetables are our life angels. Consider them the basis of your diet. Increase their consumption the most possible, try to enjoy them slowly. If you can become a vegetarian, you will reach food excellence, and you will discover great benefits for your life and that you ever imagined.

Pay attention to the wrong food association of different food classes to have the best results from the first weeks. To mix foods that are at odds with each other increases the duration of digestion, and it poisons your body. Study and study in-depth what are proteins, carbohydrates, vegetables, fruits, and dried fruits so that you have a clear and complete picture of what you put on your table.

To talk about wrong foods associations that cause body dysfunctions and to think to memorize a long list of food to avoid it, it can be scary.

In reality, it is simpler than you think

Essentials points to remember are five:

1 - Avoid mixing different proteins among them

2 - Avoid associating carbohydrates and proteins

3 - Avoid associating carbohydrates, proteins, and fats

4 - Vegetables, it's good anytime anyway

5 - Fruits must be eaten far from meals and always avoiding to associate different kinds of fruits.

Benefits of this practice are:

- ✓ Digestion is perfect, and so nutrients are absorbed without making the body heavier, and by avoiding the accumulation of fats.

✓ The purification process is helped

✓ You lose extra weight easily

✓ The body has more energy to be used.

Let's try to go to depth about that, trying to understand why the association of foods that are at odds with each other, create severe problems to digestion about gastrointestinal disorders such as abdominal swellings, long and difficult digestions, constipation and heartburn. We often believe that it's enough to stop the consumption of meat or replace refined whole-grain cereal or to choose honey instead of sugar and others. They are almost all baseless solutions. All classes are digested in different ways and times. In the digestive process, a lot of enzymes are involved, each one can act in one particular chemical bond.

Some enzymes are active in acid environments, others in an alkaline environment.

Therefore it's clear that if you put together two not suitable classes, you affect the digestion of one or the other, and you make the process more cumbersome.

For example proteins need an acid environment so that stomach will produce more hydrochloric acid to digest them. Carbohydrates are pre-digested when they are in the mouth so that in the stomach, they need an alkaline environment. If in the stomach you have an acid environment or proteins, the alkaline secretion for carbohydrates is blocked. They wait for hours to pass into the small intestine to be digested by pancreatic juices in the right alkaline environment.

What does it mean practically? It means that pasta topped with meat sauce "ragu'" lengthen the process, and it can cause abdominal swellings and fermentation. This meal is made of pasta and meat: carbohydrates and proteins topped with a vegetable fruit such as tomatoes.

Imagine what happens when you eat a well-seasoned pasta together with a second raw meat dish, a cake, fruits, and everything washed with good wine!. It's better to choose a large first dish of pasta with a glass of wine and a large salad. Next, you select meat.

PROTEIN FOOD WITH DIFFERENT PROTEIN FOOD

Usual in the same dish, we find two or more protein food of different origins. It can be a piece of cheese at the end of the meal after you ate meat or fish, or elaborate dishes such as meatloaf problem in these cases is that our stomach produces different gastric juices at different times according to the kind of protein to be digested.

One of the worse food combinations is milk and meat. Milk in contact with the acidity of stomach, clots, holding inside pieces of poorly digested and unchanged meat that go to the intestine.

As I said before in the four rules, it' enough to know proteins and to avoid eating all of them together.

BEVERAGES AND ACID FOOD WITH AMIDACE FOOD

The starches such as bread, pasta, rice, potatoes, begin to be digested in the mouth in an alkaline environment if it's matched with an acid drink that makes the environment acidic. They can go directly to the stomach while they are still structured and almost indigestible.

Lemon, vinegar, acid fruits such as pineapple, cherries, strawberries, fruit juices should be eaten far from carbohydrates. The most acid beverages are absolutely the carbonated black ones such as coke and company. These should be avoided.

BEVERAGES AND ACID FOOD WITH PROTEINS FOOD

Proteins are digested in an acid environment, so that could make us think that they are not much different from the acidity of drinks. In reality, it is exactly the opposite. The secretion of hydrochloric acid in the stomach is regulated by a mechanism: the hydrochloric acid which activates pepsin enzyme that is responsible for proteins digestion, it's only partially secreted, if the stomach environment is already acidic because it is replaced by other acids that we eat; pepsin secretion stops. Proteins are only partially digested, choking the stomach and duodenum. Proteins are digested in small parts, clogging the stomach and duodenum.

SUGAR AND FRUITS WITH AMIDACEOUS FOOD AND PROTEINS.

Sweet food such as sugar and its derivatives inhibit gastric secretion and mobility of stomach, making digestion of other classes very difficult.

Fruits need a particular mention aside. Its composition, based on simple sugars, doesn't necessarily start digesting from the mouth, they go to the small intestine, where they are directly absorbed.

If fruits are eaten alone, the time of digestion is short, if we eat it together with other classes, it must wait for the digestion of all other food before being absorbed by the small intestine. The result is that it stays in the stomach for a long time. It creates a fermentation that involves other food too.

FATS WITH PROTEIN FOOD

To eat meat, fish, eggs, butter, or cream slow down the digestive process. Fats Inhibit the acid secretion in the stomach and slow its mobility too. It happens the same with oil but to a lesser extent. If you consider the rules about the right food combinations, you can understand how it could alter our digestion when we stand up from the table after we eat what is considered a normal meal for many people: a dish of pasta, meat, and side dish, fruits, and even a little bit of cheese and a little cake to make our appetite happy. We can eat all, but when we choose some classes, we must pay attention and act with due caution and knowledge.

There are some classes we must pay attention to more than others.

As far as the first times are concerned, I have worked out a very simple trick that will help you to solve this problem.

Then with time, it will be spontaneous to study and better understand how to work with the food you eat. But use this "magic wand" to start your way.

Aside, you will find a very clear, simple, and **practical table** to have different food combinations to create and enjoy.

Really bad combination

CARBOHIDRATES

- Cereals (also pasta and bread)
- Potatoes
- Peanuts
- Corn
- Peas
- Legumes
- Lentils
- Pumpkin
- Parsnip
- Beet
- Carrots
- Artichokes
- Coconut

FAT

- Derived oils (olive, sesame, sun flower)
- Butter
- Ceram
- Cheese

- Oily fruit
- Avocado
- Seeds
- Dried fruit

PROTEIN

- Meat
- Fish
- Legumes
- Lentils
- Peas
- Egg
- Milk
- Joghurt
- Tofu
- Tempeh
- Seeds (pumpkin, sesame,....)
- Dried Fruit (nuts, almond, pistachios)

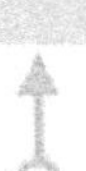
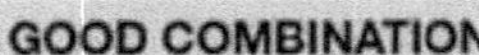
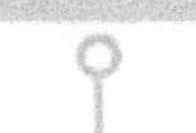

GOOD COMBINATION

GOOD COMBINATION

GOOD COMBINATION

Eat food containing many complex carbohydrates only with salad and/or

FRUIT AND VEGETABLES

Eat food containing many concentrated proteins only with

- Asparagus
- Broccoli
- Brussels Sprouts
- Cabbage
- Chinese Cabbage
- Cauliflower

- Chinese Vegetables (bok choi, sucy choi)
- Cucumber
- Aubergine
- Salad
- Koirabi

- Peppers
- Radishes
- Onion, Leek
- Celery
- Alpha-Alpha

Tomato: sour fruit vegetable without sugars. You can match it with proteins and fats but not with complex carbohydrates

FRUIT

Eat fruit always on an empty stmach

ACID
- Orange
- Lemon
- Pineapple
- Kiwi
- Strawberries
- Raspberries
- Bluebarries
- Blackbarries
- Tangerine
- Pomegranate

SWEET
- Banana
- Dates
- Dried Figs
- Raicin
- Dried Fruit

MELON
Eat melon and watermelon alone or after 10 min before other fruit

SEMI SWEET FRUIT
- Apple
- Pear
- Persimmon
- Fresh Figs
- Mango
- Grape
- Peach
- Apricot
- Cherimuya
- Papaya
- Cherrie

"About politics .. Do we have something to eat?"

Antonio de Curtis

Chapter 13

WHAT YOU SHOULD AVOID LIKE THE PLAGUE

All that is white is dangerous apart from fruits and vegetables.

White color belongs to not easily digestible food. Think about ham fat or cream, fats in animal food such as pork meat. You should eat pasta bread and different kind of flours carefully, paying attention to quantity and their associations. Milk and its derivatives, such as cheeses, must be consumed carefully and mildly.

Sugar needs a chapter aside. If you can, do not use it in your diet or change it with honey or other natural sweeteners such as stevia. Limit consumption the best way possible. Refined sugar is the first enemy of our life. I'll give you an example of how it is used in the dietary field.

In the USA, sugars are one of the major sources of calories for nutrition. The increase in sugar consumption is amazing in the last 300 years.

-1700 the yearly consumption per capita was 1.8 KG (3.9 lb)

-1800 the yearly consumption per capita was 8 KG (17.6 lb)

-1900 the yearly consumption per capita increased to 40 Kg (88.1 lb)

-2009 the yearly consumption per capita was in the average more than 80 KG (176.3 lb)

From 3 cases of diabetes on 100.000 people, they reached 8.000 cases on 100.000 people at the end of the 80s.

From the 80s to nowadays, we go from 3.4% of obese people to 32%. We should add to this 33% of overweight people. We are talking about 65% of people out of ideal weight.

It means that 2/3 of the people living in the industrialized countries actually run the risk of serious diseases and must resort to nutritionists, nutritious diets, gyms, medical care drugs, and they are often dangerous.

Nowadays, there are many sugar-free products in the market, they can help us to avoid this harmful substance. **LWBE** suggests to avoid sugar the most and to control always the content on the labels, by using the dietary tables reported on the products in the carbohydrate section with the writing "of which sugars":

In the United States Food and drug administration (FDA), the agency that regulates the alimentary and pharmaceutical sector has set a cap on the consumption of sugars: 50 grams (0.11 lb) daily, more or less the quantity contained in one can of dark beverage. FDA would like to clarify precisely this aspect, by writing on the labels the quantity of added natural sugars.

Who respects the cap of 50 grams (0.11 lb) daily consumes 10% of daily calories in the form of sugar.

The world health organization has released the new lines; according to them, children and adults should reduce the use of sugar even to less than 10% of daily calories, bringing the quantity of sugar to less than 5% and so around 25 grams (0.05 lb) in a day.

They studied that this quantity of sugar could be healthy for us too. Also, the world health association pointed its finger against added sugars hidden in processed food.

Sugar means both monosaccharides such as glucose and fructose, and disaccharides added to food produced by consumers or producers, and natural sugars that are in the honey too.

They exclude sugars present in fruits and fresh vegetables and those in milk.

We have already said that a diet rich in simple and complex sugars can cause obesity and overweight, then metabolic diseases such as diabetes hypercholesterolemia, hypertriglyceridemia but also less serious pathologies as cavity and sugar dependency from products with much quantity of sugar.

To avoid all this, it is important to know the classes which contain excessive doses, by paying attention to the labels. Apart from all cakes and sugar that we put in coffee or milk, pasta, bread, and their derivatives also contain sugars. Some ailments far from white color contain a large quantity of it, such as ketchup, mayonnaise, sweet and sour sauce, tomato paste, ready sauces, cereal bars, and so on.

We should reduce sweets and snacks, candies fizzy drinks, and already sweetened and packaged drinks.

Let's choose fresh fruits, natural yogurt, juices, and homemade drinks. Pay attention to the use of alcohol too, they bring a good quantity of simple sugars: a little glass of limoncello contains around 10 grams (0.02 lb) of sugar. Think that a can of cola fizz drink contains around 10 spoons of sugar it means: 39 grams (0.08 lb). Inside this beverage, there are other ingredients studied show that in one hour, causes severe body derangement and almost pathological addiction to the product.

We have already talked about it. Let's see what happens when we drink a 33 cl (11 oz) can of coke.

In the first 10 minutes, 39 grams (0.08 lb) of sugar enter in your system. Practically with only a can, you cover 100% of suggested daily quantity. We can avoid trow out only because the phosphoric acid contained in the can changes the very sweet flavor of beverage, this allows for swallowing it.

After 20 minutes, the sugar in the blood reaches the peak and causes a surge of insulin. The liver answers to this state by changing each possible sugar into fat. It is right here that you start to accumulate. 40 minutes after you drink it, it happens the total absorption of caffeine around 200 mg (0.0004 lb), more than a cup of coffee. The pupils are dilated, blood pressure increases and the liver dumps more sugars into the circulatory system. A great part of them is changed to fats one more time.

Receptors for adenosine in your brain are active now to fight sleepiness. 45 minutes after, the body increases the production of dopamine and stimulates pleasure centers that are in the brain.

Physically it's the same procedure activated by heroin. It is in those minutes that you develop the pathological addiction to this substance. 60 minutes later phosphoric acid ties together calcium, magnesium, and zinc in your intestine, it speeds up the metabolism. The high doses of sugars upgrade the urinary calcium secretion. Diuretic properties of caffeine start their function, and the body excretes calcium, magnesium, and zinc that were destined for the bones. A soon as the excitement decreases, a glycemia collapse occurs, you become irritable and apathetic. At this point, all water contained in the can have been excreted through urine, before the body could absorb the useful nutrients that you need to keep your system hydrated or to make strong bones and teeth; therefore, the more you drink, the more you start a slow dehydration process. Coke beverage and their counterparts are studied to create these chemical processes in our body to make it a slave. Keep in mind that to consume sugar in immoderate quantity, it means to exceed 25/30 grams (0.05/0.06 lb) per day, has the same dramatic. We said that when we will see the white color, we will pay attention to it and we will think very carefully about what to do. Is it simplistic? Yes it is, but at the very beginning, it helps.

Then, over time, you can deepen the nutrition topic to be aware of and become an expert. The white color trick is very nice, instructive, and instant. It communicates instantly that this food requires attention and certain moderation. You can eat absolutely a nice dish of pasta topped with a tasty sauce, but be careful with the quantity, chew it as long as possible, and above all, do not eat it every day. Maybe you can alternate it with another delicious dish but less white. When it is hidden among other colors, you should find it out, and you know perfectly how to do it. Your body speaks to you, and in front of a sweet pastry topped with cream, certainly, it will tell you that it's dangerous. That is an alarm. Then it's up to you. Do you want to eat it? Go ahead but chew it at least 40 times. Then the rest you already know. You start the LWBE program. Come on!

You control your goodies and body, and after 30 days, everything will be different and easier. The joy that will burn inside you, will always help to face everything with more energy and determination.

Salt or sodium chloride is an essential mineral for the human body, if it is taken through food, it helps to regulate the balance of liquids inside the body naturally. However, unregulated consumption can cause problems. One of the most common effects is the rise of water retention, particularly of the abdominal band and legs. The effects of reduced or failed drainage of liquids can be numerous and different; they can go from generalized swelling sensation with an increase and worsening of orange peel skin, to more severe problems such as edemas, hypertension, and increased risk factors for the cardiovascular system. The reduction of the assumption through diet is the preventive measure to control water retention. To adopt a diet that provides the reduction allowed to obtain quick and significant benefits both for the health and the body. The right dose of salt to stay healthy and with ideal weight is around 100-600 mg of sodium daily, it means 0.25-1.5 grams (0.008-0.05 oz) of salt per day.

Italian diet has, on average, almost 12 grams of salt daily exceeding the real necessity ten times.

Starting from these numbers, the simple reduction of salt in the diet to 6 grams (0.2 oz) daily, permits to reduce the blood pressure of 2-8 mmHg:

In Summertime, when we sweat more, it grows the need for sodium, above all for sportsmen. In a balanced diet, we recommend taking less than 6 grams of salt per day. To stay in this limit, it's necessary to pay attention to its presence inside the different products we bring on the table. Sodium is naturally present in many meals, many of them have a greater quantity in comparison with others... In nutritional tables, these measures are normally reported in milligrams -mg per portion. To get used to the attitude to verify these indications could be of great help to respect the recommended daily dose, by keeping the consumption within a maximum of 200 mg (7 oz) per portion. The same importance is to know hidden sources of sodium chloride, which are in richer food to handle consumption knowingly.

Live in various light and balanced diet.

On the Internet or TV, there are plenty of chefs and cooking programs. Let yourself be inspired by your taste and maybe put yourself in front of the stove and prepare dishes you like.

Remember, cooking for others makes hunger pass! Try!

Try to always eat light and different from the day before. A variety of food will make meals happy and exciting. I recommend small portions to respect food combination and to chew, chew, and chew...

 When you eat outside, a half well-chewed portion will be enough until dinner.

Another important topic is fasting. I'll give you a simple example.

Fasting means that if you are not hungry at lunchtime you can skip the meal. You will eat later... maybe. If at dinner time you feel full because during the day you followed **LWBE** diet, drink a herb tea and go to bed. To sleep a whole night with a "light" stomach is the best care to feel good the next day and to lose fat! Remember that your body gets used to these very quickly, above all, if the improvements better our life.

Furthermore, for strong and enterprising people, I suggest one day of fasting in a month and total relaxation. You can have only water and maximum a honey spoon and relax. After you will find yourself in paradise, you will feel purified and full of energy. It usually works in this way: 1 day fasting 1 kilo less. However, as well as feeling much better in the body, the greater benefit will be the mental one. You will discover that to stay without eating, gives to our inner life unexpected security, even if for a short time. Many people often believe that to have a big belly means to be fat. Try to tap your belly with your fingers. The better area is the right one at the high of the navel; if you hear a noise similar to a thud of a drum, which reminds of space, it means you are swollen. It means that your intestine is full of air, stagnated food, and other substances, from time.

I'll say to you their name, to let you keep your inner peace!

You have done the wrong food association for many months. To be swollen and fat, it's worse, but you can solve these situations by time. **LWBE** is a miracle. The first step to do it is to wonder if you drink sparkling beverages such as legendary coke a& friends or beer, sparkling wine, or sparkling water. Then control if you are eating foods that conflict with each other, or with food intolerances that you discovered in your initial check-up. To eat unsuitable food for our body has unimaginable consequences because certain habits are longstanding and our body is overwhelmed for a long time. What is dramatic is that we think we are eating properly and that there are few alternatives to junk food we're eating daily. There is no alternative to the way we eat. **LWBE** creates a healthy diet from all points of view, both physical and mental.

It sets up completely new attitudes that change those that operate in our life in an unhealthy way. Another very important item to be considered is your excretion pace. Usually, 15-30 days are enough to have a nutritional way that borders on perfection. Water, movement, and digestion that starts with a well-chewed bolus create smooth paths and purify the body totally from toxins.

WHAT TO DO IN NEXT PERIOD

Set up a monthly plan where you eliminate or slowly reduce the four white poisons.

SUGAR

SALT

FLOUR

MILK

" We all need to believe in something... I believe that in a while I'll have a beer "

Homer Simpson

Chapter 14

DON'T EAT LESS, EAT CONSCIOUSLY! ... AND HOW TO DO IT

You Don't Have to Eat Less, You Just Have to eat Right ✔

Keeping in mind what is said until now, we can talk about how to create healthy food attitudes. As we have already said in previous chapters many times, **LWBE** is a method that makes positive habits for our body and permits us to eat and live in the best way, by bringing back to us our ideal weight. Finally it gives us that happiness that comes from being healthy.

This method is based principally on the way to swallow food and on the creation of digestion as perfect as possible. This means to assimilate only the necessary food, without useless accumulations. **LWBE** tries to bring back our food habits as they were hundreds of years ago. It braces its positive value through modern scientific studies. In this way, we obtain a diet that leads our life to get the maximum from food, without weighing down and consequently not getting fat.

It tries to bring us to our ideal weight, and it always succeeds. The method is foolproof.

As we said, in the beginning, it gives us only suggestion to eat in the best way possible. One of the best methods to help our body and our life to reach the maximum of its potential is to eat predominantly vegetables, fruits, legumes, and whole wheat. According to my modest opinion, the best way in absolute is to choose and become vegetarian slowly, by following studies and scientific plans that help to start this important step. I try to limit the use of animal meat as much as possible;

but I believe that to eat without any mental complications, is much more important than studies and deprivation, in this world where being a vegetarian is very difficult.

I discovered an alimentary food program based on blood groups. It is excellent for my body and my personality. However, I slightly turn to vegetarian feeding because it is less intoxicating and gives much more energy both physically and mentally.

Diet based on blood groups takes into consideration the choice of food, recipes, quantities, and times to be eaten. It steers only to the assumption of certain products based on people's blood group. Let's discover together its basis and function that is perfectly suitable to **LWBE** .

A blood group diet was conceived by Peter d'Adamo, a naturopathic doctor. He believes that blood group A B and 0 is the first topic to be considered to create a healthy diet. The reasoning is based on a perfectly sociological-anthropological observation. The primary blood group of humanity belongs to 0. It was the only one until all the world was populated.

Group A Type

Comes from a mutation that happened in the place and moment when man became sedentary, becoming a farmer. Studies certify this place to be in the fertile crescent area.

Group B Type

Comes from a mutation that occurred in the areas where agriculture was limited, because of environmental conditions, such as Tibet and Siberia, so that man was forced to become cattle breeders.

Group AB Type

It is very rare, comes from a very recent mutation around a thousand years ago. It comes from the genetic cross of A and B. These analyses rely on the territorial distribution of different groups.

Diet conclusions are: GROUP o has hunter and gatherer features, group A farmer features group B cattle breeder, group AB farmer, and cattle breeder, diet is based exactly on these attitudes.

The idea of feeding, according to the blood group arises from the need to understand why people react differently to the same diet. For example why what is good for someone, is bad for another?

The answer is in the immune system, which is strictly connected to the blood group. Our immune system detects the " intruders" in the body thanks to substances called antigens; they have two functions:

1) Monitoring service

2) They define blood groups themselves.

Once they identify harmful substances, they communicate with cells through a simple sugar chain. Their alarm stimulates the production of antibodies. The key to the connection between food and the immune system are lectins, a particular family of proteins contained in foods. All lectins react differently to single antigens. When they find an "unintelligible" one, agglutination starts, cells bind together and create lumps that in part will be excreted trough urinary system and feces and in part, they will be deposited on the walls of internal organs, by causing inflammations that could be less or more serious depending on the degree of compatibility. Doctor d'Adamo verified scientifically the effects of lectins in different blood groups. He examined all the most ordinary ailments, and he texted their compatibility with different blood groups creating an alimentary diet.

It is a diet that has few deprivations and used together with **LWBE** gives the possibility to eat studied aliments for our blood group in the best way possible. I feel very comfortable, and I suggest it to all people that choose our diet.

A blood group diet is very tasty and easy to follow. Above all, it gives us the security to eat suitable food to our blood personality, by avoiding complications and food inflammations.

I believe that to associate this scientific study with the rules of food combination and **LWBE** is the best nutritional technique you can have.

During the years, the man had to fit to weather environmental and food conditions. These adjustments allow him to survive, but they have also provoked great changes in the immune system, by creating a diversification of antigens in the blood.

Neanderthal men were inexperienced predators, they ate wild plants grubs and animals killed by other predators.

40.000 years ago, at the time of Cro-Magnon man, our ancestors that belonged to group 0 became hunters, they ate meat principally. They were at the pole position of the alimentary chain. They moved from Europe to Asia to find out new hunting territories.

After 30.000 years, they reached all parts of the planet by populating   it.
Nowadays, group 0 is still the most common in the world. During the neolithic age, the first important change occurred: the nomadic man became sedentary. In Asia and the middle east the first agricultural communities were born, it was based on cereals cultivation and cattle breeding. The population along the rivers or the seaside practiced fishing. In this new environment, it started to develop group A, that nowadays it is principally concentrated in the Mediterranean area. The gene of B group appears in the nomadic populations of Asia, that moved in the mountain areas of the country 10.000 years ago. It was born to face the transition from the torrid climate of Africa to the glacial cold of Himalaya. These populations devoted to herding; consequently, they ate only meat and cheese products. This culture

spreads in Europe, to date, can be found in Germany, China, and Southeast Asia. Another percentage of B group is present in the Jewish population. The anthropologists are not sure about the dynamic that caused this phenomenon.

Finally, group AB is the most recent as well as the most uncommon of everyone. It is present in less than 5% of the population. Its appearance dates back around 1000-1200 years ago when the Roman Empire was raided by barbarians and blood type A mixed with type B.

It is difficult to know exactly in which period it happened, but studies about remains discovered in Hungary, show without any doubts that blood group AB was not present in the Lombard period (IV-VII century A.C.)

This blood group presents complex and contradictory characteristics: It inherits tolerances of both groups, but it has antibodies of none of them; this makes it resistant and vulnerable at the same time.

Group O Type

It is the oldest group:

It belongs to the first men that got food by hunting. People belonging to group o has a very reactive immune system. The digestive system is very strong and has an internal acid environment that can tolerate a slight state of ketosis. That is an alteration of metabolism due to a diet that is very rich in proteins and fats and poor in carbohydrates. This helps to metabolize the animal aliments at best. To be healthy, it needs a diet rich in animal proteins, vegetables, legumes matched to a strong physical activity program. It tolerates very little quantity of legumes because its organism is not suitable for this kind of ailment.

Group O must pay attention to gluten: its lectins interfere with metabolism by weakening the activity of insulin, and this causes weight gain, in time, it can reach serious diseases such as diabetes. Who belongs to this group, reacts to stress in a very fast and instinctive way, exactly as its ancestor hunters, that were forced to react quickly in dangerous situations. Stress effects focus on muscles. The best way to release stress is to practice strong physical exercises such as aerobics, rope, weightlifting, martial arts, jogging, swimming, tapis roulant, step, rhythmic gymnastics, bike (or cycle) walking, dance, and skating. Every person belonging to o group has in his genetic memory: strength, endurance sense of self-esteem, recklessness, intuition, and optimism. These qualities are perfectly suitable to their hostile environment. Other observed characteristics of this group are the inclination to success and qualities to become a leader, many people that played a powerful role in the world belong to group 0, such as the majority of Japanese prime ministers.

Group A: it developed after the born of first agricultural communities

It is characterized by a sensible immune system and by infections.

A healthy diet for people belonging to group A is made principally of fruits, vegetables, fish, and eggs.

Group A is almost the opposite of group 0. Their digestive system is not too acidic, does not tolerate ketosis. It assimilates red meat badly, which is stored as fat. Dairy products are not tolerated too, and they can slow metabolism. People belonging to group A are very sensitive to stressful situations, above all mentally talking. Adrenaline gives stress, and it affects the nervous system principally. This phenomenon causes them to be anxious and irritable. The best way to face it is to start a physical activity that promotes mental relaxation, such as yoga, Thai chi, Chuan, quick walking, martial arts, golf, swimming, dance, aerobic exercises (light), and stretching.

Group A preserves the genetic inheritance of first farmers of history. They were also the first human beings that organized themselves in a community, learning to cooperate, and to respect the times of nature to obtain agricultural products to eat. Furthermore, they had to be socially acceptable, tidy, sensible, intuitive, respectful of the law, and to have good self-control.

For that reason, people belonging to group A tend to have a stronger emotional structure, and they preserve psychological traits that give them a great ability to plan and cooperate.

They can be good leaders, but they refuse to have any excessively aggressive behaviors to fulfill their role.

Group B: This group comes from ancient nomadic tribes in Asia that had to fit the mountain climate.

Group B's immune system is resistant to many pathologies but liable to autoimmune diseases and those with slow-growing viruses: such as multiple sclerosis and lupus. People belonging to this group can follow a very varied diet because their digestive system is very suitable for feeding changes. B people, if able to maintain a balance between body and mind, handle stress very well. When this capacity fails, bothers can arise, such as chronicle wearing and mental clouding. The best physical activities for them are those that involve both body and mind slightly, swimming, foot or bike excursions, aerobic, tennis, martial arts, slight rope, rhythmic gym, quick walking, jogging, weights lifting, golf, and yoga.

B kind people's password is "balance." This group belonged genetically to nomadic conquerors, that had to be flexible and creatives. They can examine each situation, putting themselves in others' shoes so that they live and act with empathy. In Asia, group B is very well represented Chinese traditional medicine considers a perfect physical emotive and psychical balance to be healthy.

Group AB

It is the most recent and rare blood group. It was born from the mix of groups A and B. It has characteristics similar to both of them. The immune system is resistant to infectious diseases, thanks to the presence of both antigens. It is characterized by the lack of antibody anti-A and anti-B. This represents both an advantage and a drawback; from aside, it is more resistant to allergies and other immune diseases, on the other hand, it identifies with more difficulty foreign cells that are allied to Group A and B. Digestive system has a very high tolerance. However, it also has the poor acidity of group A, this makes the digestion of red meat difficult. Furthermore, it has some intolerance of group B to corn, buckwheat, sesame, and wheat. They reduce insulin efficiency.

As far as stress management is concerned, it is similar to group A. Adrenalin acts on the nervous system, it gives an emotive reaction principally tending to anxiety and irritability.

Physical activity which helps to relax is the best solution, such as, Yoga, Quick Walking, Light Rope, Taichi, Chuan, Aikido, Golf, Bike, Swimming, Dance, Aerobic (light), Foot Excursions, Stretching. According to these studies, the personality of the AB group people is represented from the mix between the sensibility of group A and the balance of group B. The result is original persons that are very sensitive to the most spiritual side of existence. Sometimes they are impulsively endowed of great charisma and confidence in others. It is incredibly alarming to think that food changed our ancestor's needs in a thousand years, and in the last fifty hundred years, we completely upset our feeding worldwide.

We turned worryingly to food production based almost entirely on chemistry and profit logic. This annihilates resoundingly the collective awareness that wants to have healthy and tasty products on their tables. The food market was built horribly. Third world countries starving, while in developed ones food is thrown into the garbage, 30% of created food, each day.

In the last 20 years, meat commerce has progressively increased. Once, it was healthy and valuable. Nowadays, it creates numerous animal breeding. They are fed with food mixed with chemical substances such as antibiotics and anti-inflammatory; they guarantee animal health until its dramatic slaughter. Tolstoj wrote: If slaughterhouses had glass walls, we would be all vegetarians. Precisely because of this modern idea, which creates chemical food only to earn money and to our detriment, many people turned gradually to eat only vegetable products; this avoids the killing of any being. Frankly speaking, I must say that I consider being vegetarian a cultural conquer and a great sign of civilization. A vegetarian feels to be an earth citizen, because he respects its inhabitants, even responding to his primordial need for food. Vegetarian pride is similar to that one felt from Greeks. They belonged to the first philosophical school convinced vegetarians starting from Leonardo da Vinci to Beatles made their choice a flag. It means a certain world view: less violence, less death, more consciousness, and more sense of individual responsibility. Probably, Einstein was the first one to call Vegetarianism a necessity for human survival by connecting private food choices to the resources balance of the planet. Though, we should consider the personal attitudes of each of us for a vegetarian choice.

O Group people will have great difficulties to become vegetarians. Who wants to do that for conscience or food reasons, take it one step at a time, with a lot of prowess.

Nowadays, our survival is seriously threatened in comparison with Einstein's time.

We are 7 billion on the earth, and it is foreseen that we'll be 9 billion in 2050.

You should add to human beings 4 billion cattle that feed the already supercharged minority of people, taking away food to people that are still starving. If today we are in trouble to satisfy 7 billion of mouths that must eat and drink, we should wonder which is the limit beyond which, the catastrophic fight for food, will break out. Sure we can trust science and in its ability to increase the quantity and quality of water and food resources, but sooner or later we will reach that limit. The civil world should already ensure a future for the next generations. There is an immediate solution more acceptable and effective in effect: to limit the use of meat, Einsteins' solution. Meat is an aliment contrary to environmental sustainability. We need 15 or 20 thousand liters (3960 – 5280 gal) of water to obtain a kilogram (2.20 lb) of meat, while you need 1000 liters (264 gals) to have a kilogram of cereals. Cattle are 4 billion animals that produce carbon dioxide and consume oxygen, that steals arable lands on the earth or whole forests, which are pure air sources. Caw, fish, chickens, pigs, which are battery produced, are transported for miles until it reaches our tables. These are the consequences of intensive breeding in our health and on the planet. Therefore, to reduce the consumption of meat, is a choice that points out environmental respect and responsibility for man's future. It is, above all, a love choice for life, for animals, and us. Vegetarians already realize this reality. They do not eat meat, and they are happy and proud; who needs to limit its consumption, maybe replace it with fish or other vegetarian proteins. Many people decide to be vegetarian also to avoid the introduction of toxins and chemicals in their bodies. Others choose a sense of consciousness and animal esteem, especially for those of breeding. Think that all people say the same things and have the same results, after leaving the omnivorous diet for the vegetarian one. They feel better, they feel stronger, and above all, they are in perfect ideal weight. Who is interested in knowing and in experimenting this healthy method of eating, I'll say some words about the way to approach this wonderful world of green food.

We usually start slowly, without heads shots or drastic and sudden changes. It is better to have a road friend that already knows it and has already made the change to vegetarianism. It will help us with some useful suggestions. We must consider that to eliminate animal proteins from our body, we need the classic 30 days to fit it. Now I want to talk about another very particular aspect of the way to eat. Usually, we eat solid raw or cooked food. There is not a well-known side of LWBE to the rest of the feeding world. It helps in an excellent way of food absorption. When you prepare a dish, pay close attention to the wrong food associations. When a dish is ready, try to whisk food. Whisk different food portions, separately, to give back to food its tenderness which they had before being cut (lightly dehydrated), add a little bit of oil, water or broth spoon, and if the recipe permits a bit of excellent wine. Then hit it. It will come out with a delicious, very delicious cream. Work it until it comes out as velvet. To change it into a bolus, you must eat it in the same way you eat solid food. In this case, this transition from whisked food to bolus happens only through the spittle secretion, which will permeate the morsel through mouth movements.

Swallowing time is different according to food. Sometimes a bit is so good that we would like it to stay always in our mouth. Ptyalin works out faster, the liquid cream permeates bolus more deeply. The result is that food reaches the stomach ready to be digested without much effort, our body feels full much before. It takes from it the maximum of energies. By the time, you will be able to do it the best way possible. It will be a wonderful discovery that will be with you all your life. This way to eat seems to be crazy, but think about when we taste asparagus or mushrooms cream or soup, we do the same thing, and we taste delicious food. The method is foolproof.

"Each time I say to my self this will be the last time, but then I smell that chocolate flavor… chocolate shells! So little, so simple, so innocent. I thought: oh only a little bit can do nothing bad, then I discovered they were filled with rich sinful… And it melts, God forgives me, it melts so slowly in your mouth, and it fills you with pleasure."

Jonny Deep (from the movie Chocolate)

Chapter 15

ADVICE TO CHANGE YOUR ERRONEOUS HABITS

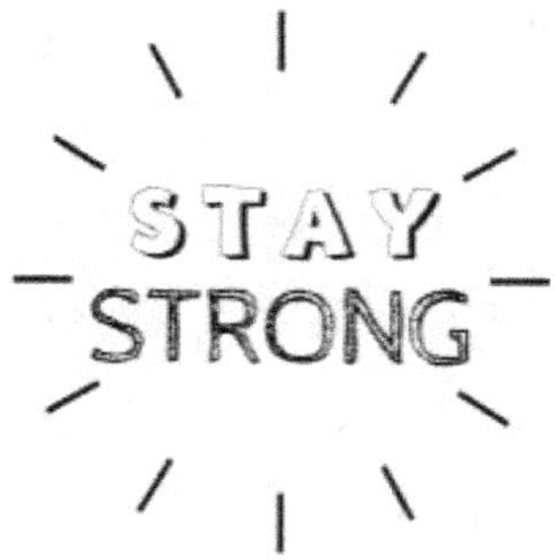

First **LWBE** times are the most difficult to find a balance between learning and practicing the new attitudes, to understand what to eat and which food to avoid. It is complicated for everybody. As far as each enterprise is concerned, we need some will to face the first steps slightly and slowly, by focusing on constancy. To give energy to **LWBE** and to have the charge, I suggest you do this: In the first month every 20 days, you allow yourself a few tears to the rule. You go to a restaurant, and you order your favorite dishes, or you cook and prepare them by yourself. Then you sit at the table, and you taste everything and how you want to.

However, my suggestion is to eat slowly, to chew, and to limit yourself in portions.

The program will help you to get used to it. To suddenly overcharge the digestive system is unhealthy. This is useful, above all, to feel morally good and to feel that the joy and enthusiasm to be greedy, is deprived of old habits. It is recommended to eat fried food, at least once a month, maybe fish. If you overstate at a table, the day after will be such as you are waking up from a happy state. You will feel weighed down, dazed, and accepting. Start again eat lightly, and within 24 hours, you will feel as before; if somebody exaggerates with tears to the rules, good for him. To overstate means a great laugh together, breaking the monotony. It is done with no excesses and only to be happy.

There are people affected by bulimia, this is a consequence of uncontrollable food disruptions. It is about problems due to internal imbalances; often, they come from childhood or are caused by organic diseases. In case you have to face these problems, I heartily recommend you talk to your doctor to handle the situations together with trusted practitioners, to work on yourself about this issue calmly and confidently, before starting the diet. I would like to underline the word trusted, to avoid some kind of doctors that listen, listen, and listen to you without talking. After one year, they say to you: " Your father personality has made a great impact on your deep unconscious.. bla bla.." In the meantime, they take 100 bucks for a weekly session. I suggest you talk to a person freely and that in each session helps you to understand, to react, and plan. In this life, everything can be solved, be sure of that. These problems, which involve many people, can be settled because there are already tested and successfully conducted practices. The best strategy is to do a complete check-up, as suggested at the beginning, then go to a psychologist or a psychiatrist with your right body value in your hands to start to work on reliable data. Often, we think wrongly that there are mental implications, but in reality, it is only our body that works in the wrong way. I saw fat, confused, and depressed people doing medical check-up only to discover hypothyroid. The dark tunnel, where they were walking in their desperate life, was only caused by the lack of a substance normally excreted from a glad, located at the base of the throat. As soon as they discovered the right quantity of levothyroxine hormone secreted by the thyroid, they started to smile again. They began a diet, and they reached their once ideal weight after one year.

I can give you thousands of examples.

The message is:

STAY Strong !

YOU Can Do It !

YOU Will Do It !

Trust yourself...

drink, sweat, and chew... always.

*"A day should start with a hug, a kiss, a caress,
and a coffee because breakfast should be plentiful"*

Charles Shulz (peanuts)

Chapter 16

SILENCE IS GOLD !

shhh

This LWBE is very important. It needs a strong will and no mercy. Try to be always faithful to this: silence is gold.

For the first month, tell nobody you are doing **LWBE**. It is essential to be silent and discreet for this first time. Then when you get used to this healthy lifestyle, and you know the method perfectly, you can start to suggest it to those people around you that you love, carefully, and confidentially but always without waving it to the four winds. Eventually, you can take care of them without being too invasive, so that they can create their food diet in the best way. The first month of **LWBE** is like a baby, you have to protect and pampered it. It is like meeting your first love, the bells ring in your head. You fly 5 meters from the earth, many people realize it, and they make you answer thousands of questions. Will you say anything about it to any of them? I'm sure that you will talk little even with the dearest person around you. You will say only a little bit of it, but only to the most intimate people. Here you are working on your life, your happiness. Do your own business.

The world is full of people talking about that great nutritionist that last year gave them a customized diet, and they lost 15 kilograms (33 lb) in 60 days. Then take a look at them and you see that they are 155 cm (61 in) tall and weigh 74 kilos (163 lb)! If you tell your secret to somebody, you run a great risk. You talk to injured people, and when they listen to the various rules you follow, they will start to refuse and denigrate them. They will confuse your certainties, and they will take away your inner strength. In reality, you need to be nurtured, because you are working on yourself, and you listen to these "mythological examples." Dejection takes over, almost always. On the other hand, there are envious people, when they see you're losing weight and they see a new light on your face and you are much more beautiful they ask you: " What have you done?" You are really in great shape! A soon as they hear that you discovered Idm and you are learning its rules, they start to say: " You are doing it all wrong, 30 days to get used to it is a big lie !" and so on, until they will say " my nutritionist gave me a personalized diet, and I lost 15 kilos (33 lb) in 60 days!" You watch them, you bite your lips because you revealed your secret to them and they destroyed it, by taking away your strength and trust. The worse is that they are always the same people, 155 cm (61 in) tall, and weigh 74 kilos (163 lb)!. You think to be right and to be understood by people that share the same problems with you. In reality, who is in front of you sees you slimmer, beautiful, and happy. They remember exactly that when they were under a diet, they would have eaten nutritionists too; after a few months of deprivations and rejections, they failed their goal abjectly to lose weight. After a while, they find themselves worse than before. What were you expecting from them? Good congratulations?. These poor injured people will shoot all bullets of their cannons against you to destroy you. You will win, but some bullets will take you! Why should we rescue useless snubs and disappointments? Have you never had a true secret? One of them belonging only to you? Those that give you the inner strength to preserve a treasure jealously? This should be the feeling you should have the first time. After a month or two, you will see that you can reveal your secret because in the meanwhile it will already be a part of your life. Nobody can take it away from you. Nobody can say something about you and **LWBE** because of the results that you will get, will speak for themselves; rather, they will implore you to reveal to them how you got it; then you will suggest it, by doing good to other people that need it. I hope I was clear. In the beginning, silence. I would dare to say to be silent always with your family. I ask you only 30 days of silence until **LWBE** is a part of your life; after that, everything will be easier after you can also suggest this book so that they can have paper support to read the rules and different suggestions again sometimes.

Repetita juvant (to repeat help)

" Coffee to be good must be black as the night hot as the hell and sweet as love "

Turkish saying

CONCLUSION

Drink Water !
chew !
Move !

In this final chapter, we will do a general summary to make the most important stages to practice our method clear. The first thing to do is to go to a doctor and ask for a complete checkup. Make blood tests in the best way possible. Regulate if you are celiac, and above all, check intensely if you have allergies and food intolerances. In the meantime, while you are waiting for your results, start to practice **LWBE** and prepare yourself for the future; if it is all OK in your tests choose a day and start. Remember to start calmly, slowly, and with no rush. How much time did you take to be born or start to walk? To be joyful for the first kiss or first love? Be calm to run is useless. The right road is sweetness. I talked immediately about **LWBE** because it is the core of the food diet that we should build in our life. To chew. This way, you prepare food bites to be changed to bolus. When it is in the stomach, it changes again to chimo, now it is in the best conditions to be digested. There, digestion will be simple, and the food will turn to energy without accumulating fat.

To chew food means to enjoy food; it is not a senseless stress counting. The idea is to eat lying and relaxing on a sofa, as old Romans used to do. A Japanese saying says: "stand up from your table with an almost full belly": I believe this to be one of the best strategies; following the **LWBE** program, you can eat everything, every food, chocolate too. You must only pay attention to the food match. I suggest you read about these rules again to learn them very well and by heart. Sugar has a chapter aside, but we can summarize it only in one word: delete it completely. It takes a month and much study because it is everywhere. To live without sugar means being born again!. Furthermore, before we say pay attention to white food that is principally fat and goes into thighs and legs. As far as my life is concerned, I chose to approach the diet based on blood groups. This method was studied by professor Peter D'Adamo, and I found it ingenious. Peter d'Adamo, a naturopathic doctor, says that blood group is the first aspect to be considered to make a healthy diet.

Each blood group has its ancestral characteristics. They outline different needs about nutrition and character aptitudes to follow. As far as I'm concerned, it is perfect and I'm slightly turning to the meaningful use of fruits and vegetables. Who can become vegetarian does good for himself and to nature. About other needs and food preferences, there are many more or less valid diets in the world. What is important is to follow them by practicing **LWBE**. It will help you with all and everything. I suggest you above all choose a good and testing diet such as the Mediterranean diet. A very important chapter talks about water. The highest priority to this source of life, which is the highest percentage in our body, for that reason we must renew it daily. The perfect quantity for our body is around 2 liters (0.52 gal) per day, far from meals. I recommend fish. You must increase the fish quantity that you can eat in your life, by integrating it with omega 3 capsules and by cooking it more often. Another basic rule of this book is to create the habit of moving and sweating a little. The result of healthy daily training is to increase endorphins and serotonin secretion, the so-called happiness hormones. Physical activity is more important for the secretion of these two substances than to lose weight. When joy slowly comes back to your heart, and you will train steadily, you will lose weight quickly without even realizing it. The energies you used to solve the weight problem will be directed to the creation of a new virtue: to be an active person.

A very important chapter in this book is dedicated to supplies. It was discovered that major deadly diseases of our country are caused by food lacks, instead of eaten products. This is upsetting. After different studies about this topic group: B vitamins, C vitamin, and an essential supply are strongly recommended. They bring all the necessary elements to the body daily.

This book is over. Only 4 words more that I suggest to you... to learn by heart :

DRINK, CHEW, MOVE, AND
EAT IN THE RIGHT WAY.

MANY GOOD WISHES TO YOU!

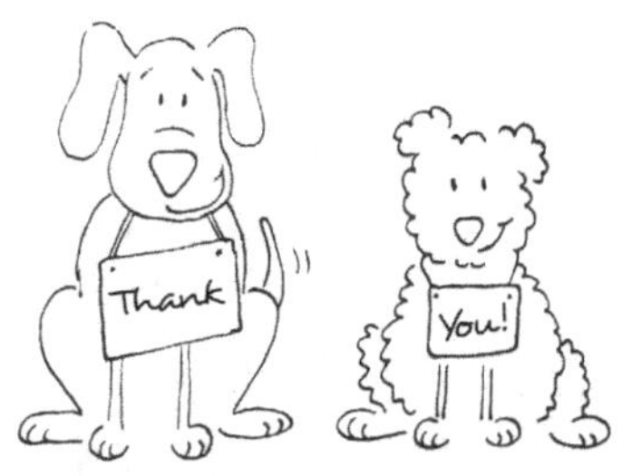

Thank You For Reading My Book!

First of all, thank you for purchasing this book. I know you could have picked any number of books to read, but you picked this book and for that I am extremely grateful.

I hope that it added value and quality to your everyday life. If so, it would be nice if you could share this book with your friends and family by posting to <u>Facebook</u> and <u>Twitter</u>.

If you enjoyed this book and found some benefit in reading this, I'd like to hear from you and hope that you could take some time to post a review on Amazon. Your feedback and support will help this author to greatly improve his writing craft for future projects and make this book even better.

Please leave a review on <u>Amazon </u>now.